THE NEW PREGNANCY

"Read this book. There is no other like it. It's honest, accurate, and forward-looking."

—Marcia Storch, M.D., Assistant Professor
of Obstetrics and Gynecology,
College of Physicians and Surgeons;
Columbia University

"The March of Dimes Birth Defects Foundation considers that the book's health, medical, and nutritional advice is so complete and up to date that it recommends that chapters around the country include the book in appropriate educational presentations."

—*American Baby*

"This unique book discusses, in depth, all the subjects that pregnant women have had difficulty getting concrete information on in the past. . . . I would highly recommend this book for all pregnant women, those who are thinking of becoming pregnant, as well as the general public."

—Kathy Wright, Co-Director of Parent Education
C/SEC (Cesareans/Support Education and Concern)

BETTER HOMES AND GARDENS® NEW BABY BOOK

CARING FOR YOUR UNBORN CHILD by Ronald E. Gots, M.D., Ph.D. and Barbara A. Gots, M.D.

CHOICES IN CHILDBIRTH by Dr. Silvia Feldman

COMPLETE BOOK OF BREASTFEEDING by Marvin Eiger, M.D. and Sally Olds

FEED ME! I'M YOURS by Vicki Lansky

THE FIRST TWELVE MONTHS OF LIFE edited by Frank Caplan

HAVE IT YOUR WAY by Vicki E. Walton

HAVING A BABY AFTER THIRTY by Elisabeth Bing and Libby Colman

IMMACULATE DECEPTION by Suzanne Arms

MAKING YOUR OWN BABY FOOD by James Turner

MAKING LOVE DURING PREGNANCY by Elisabeth Bing and Libby Colman

MOVING THROUGH PREGNANCY by Elisabeth Bing

NAME YOUR BABY by Laureina Rule

NINE MONTHS READING: A MEDICAL GUIDE FOR PREGNANT WOMEN by Robert E. Hall, M.D.

NO-NONSENSE NUTRITION FOR YOUR BABY'S FIRST YEAR by Jo-Ann Heslin, Annette B. Natow and Barbara C. Raven

PREGNANCY NOTEBOOK by Marcia Colman Morton

PREPARING FOR PARENTHOOD by Dr. Lee Salk

THE SECOND TWELVE MONTHS OF LIFE by Frank and Theresa Caplan

A SIGH OF RELIEF: THE FIRST-AID HANDBOOK FOR CHILDHOOD EMERGENCIES by Martin I. Green

SIX PRACTICAL LESSONS FOR AN EASIER CHILDBIRTH by Elisabeth Bing

UNDERSTANDING PREGNANCY AND CHILDBIRTH by Sheldon H. Cherry, M.D.

YOU *CAN* HAVE A BABY by Sherwin A. Kaufman, M.D.

YOUR BABY'S SEX: NOW YOU CAN CHOOSE by David M. Rorvik with Landrum B. Shettles, M.D., Ph.D.

THE NEW PREGNANCY

The Active Woman's Guide To Work, Legal Rights, Health Care, Travel, Sports, Dress, Sex and Emotional Well-Being

**Susan S. Lichtendorf
and
Phyllis L. Gillis**

BANTAM BOOKS
Toronto / New York / London / Sydney

THE NEW PREGNANCY

*A Bantam Book / published by arrangement with
Random House Inc.*

PRINTING HISTORY

Random House edition published October 1979
A Selection of Your Parent Book Club December 1979
Serialized in Red Book Magazine November 1979

Grateful acknowledgment is made to the following for permission to
reprint previously published material:
The American College of Obstetricians and Gynecologists: Excerpts from
Guidelines on Pregnancy and Work by The American College of Obstetri-
cians and Gynecologists.
Carol Dilfer: Excerpts from "Jogging Through Pregnancy," adapted from The
Jogger, the National Jogging Association, vol. 8, no. 36, March/April 1976.
Reprinted from The Jogger with permission of the National Jogging Associ-
ation, Washington, D.C. This later appeared in Your Baby, Your Body:
Fitness through Pregnancy, published by Crown Publishers.
Little, Brown & Company: Excerpts and adaptations from Human Sexual
Response by William Masters and Virginia E. Johnson. Copyright © 1966 by
William Masters and Virginia E. Johnson. Used by permission of Little,
Brown & Company and the authors.
McCall's Magazine: Excerpt from "What Your Obstetrician Thinks of You,"
December 1952, by Jane Whitbread and Vivian Cadden.
McGraw-Hill Book Company: Excerpt from Gynecology and Obstetrics: The
Health Care of Women, 2nd ed., by Seymour Romney, M.D., et al., 1975.
March of Dimes Birth Defects Foundation: Excerpt from pamphlet Food and
Pregnancy, published by the March of Dimes Birth Defects Foundation.
The New York Times: Excerpts from "Travel for the Pregnant, When,
Where and Whether" by Susan S. Lichtendorf, October 24, 1976. Copy-
right © 1976 by The New York Times Company. Excerpt from "Hers" by
Phyllis Theroux, September 15, 1977. Copyright © 1977 by The New
York Times Company. Reprinted by permission.

Bantam edition / August 1981

ISBN 0-553-14722-6

Published simultaneously in the United States and Canada

Bantam Books are published by Bantam Books, Inc. Its trademark, con-
sisting of the words "Bantam Books" and the portrayal of a bantam, is
Registered in U.S. Patent and Trademark Office and in other countries.
Marca Registrada. Bantam Books, Inc., 666 Fifth Avenue, New York,
New York 10103.

PRINTED IN THE UNITED STATES OF AMERICA

0 9 8 7 6 5 4 3 2 1

To our husbands and children,
who helped
from the conception

ACKNOWLEDGMENTS

With gratitude and admiration, we acknowledge a profound debt to the women who so willingly shared their personal experiences of pregnancy to help others through this book.

In addition, many generous people contributed encouragement and knowledge. Our thanks are many, and we extend them to Irwin H. Kaiser, M.D., Ph.D.; Marcia Storch, M.D.; Ivan Strausz, M.D.; John D'Urso, M.D.; Roy Pitkin, M.D.; Sidney Arje, M.D.; Sourya Henderson, Ph.D.; Sallie Schumacher, Ph.D.; Karl Rugart, M.D.; Barbara Blum, Ph.D.; Barbara Brennan, C.N.M.; Shirley Dion; Bryce Britton; Robert Mander; and Dorothy Davis.

We appreciated insights from Mark Schulman, Ph.D.; David Neft, Ph.D.; Patricia S. Cook, Ph.D.; Carol Schiro Greenwald, Ph.D.; Nicholas and Joan Tortorello; Peter Wendell; David Daines; and Gail Freilich that helped us achieve our objectives and refine our early drafts. In addition, special thanks must be offered to Louis Harris and Humphrey Taylor.

Throughout this endeavor we had the invaluable assistance of our chief researcher, Jeanne Borie. Our sincere thanks also go to Ellen Levine, Jackie Farber, Anna Monardo, Ellen Prior, Kathleen Heenan, Sandra Karp, Eva Hallman, Shirley Weiss and Linda Chesterman. We want to thank the staff of the New York Academy of Medicine library.

Finally we must thank our typists—Tom Liotta, Barbara Gilpatrick, Meryl Perlman and Asy Smith—without whom nothing would have been fit to print.

CONTENTS

INTRODUCTION

by Irwin H. Kaiser, M.D., Ph.D.
PROFESSOR OF GYNECOLOGY AND OBSTETRICS
AT THE ALBERT EINSTEIN COLLEGE OF MEDICINE
DIRECTOR, DEPARTMENT OF OBSTETRICS AND
GYNECOLOGY AT THE HOSPITAL OF THE ALBERT EINSTEIN
COLLEGE OF MEDICINE

What can possibly be new about pregnancy? Pregnancies still begin in the time-honored manner and proceed majestically to a successful conclusion 265 days later. Despite a host of technological advances, the process of labor remains essentially unchanged, and the recovery from pregnancy and labor has likewise not been altered.

What's really new about pregnancy is the woman of the present day. Although society takes many things quite for granted in its expectations of her, she no longer unquestioningly accepts the classic definitions of her role. She is in many ways the finest flower of a generation of rising expectations.

A resident in our training program recently delivered her first child after a pregnancy and labor which were in no way extraordinary. She had worked until a few days earlier. The following evening, some twenty-eight hours after this young physician's delivery, another patient was ready for delivery with a rare complication of labor. Our resident, without a word to anyone, changed from her nightgown into a surgical scrub suit and joined us in the delivery room. Clearly, having just had a baby was not going to deter this doctor from advancing her education in the care of women.

Although the present book is directed toward women like our resident, it must not be supposed that they are superwomen, from either a psychological or a physical

xi

point of view. Thirty-eight years ago, at the start of my professional experience, we confidently informed women that they could not do things which today are commonplace. After delivery, usually under general anesthesia, patients were confined to bed for a period of seven to ten days. Then, after a few days of dangling their legs over the edge of the bed, their first attempts to walk were uncertain and unsteady. Women who were perfectly healthy were thus invalided for two to three weeks by medical decisions. We did this because of our social attitudes and not because of any reliable body of scientific information.

We have since unlearned a good deal of this unnecessary baggage. The London experience in the blitz of World War II taught us early ambulation after childbirth, and we know now that healthy women can literally walk away from a normal delivery. As we adapted to the shortage of anesthesiologists during that war and the subsequent baby boom, it became clear that profound anesthesia was unnecessary for a normal birth. The need for women in the work force has made possible the demonstration that women can work until late in pregnancy.

In the background of these experiences in which we rediscovered old wisdom is the profound improvement in the safety of pregnancy, which has taken place since the turn of the century. In about 1900, the maternal mortality rate for pregnancy and childbirth was about three deaths for every hundred live births. At present it is about three for every twenty thousand, a two hundredfold decrease. The loss of infants in the early months of life has undergone a comparable drop. This has been a revolutionary and immensely liberating change. Such observations as these and many others related to them make up much of what this book has to say about pregnancy, and of course they apply to ordinary women living conventional lives and having unremarkable pregnancies.

The first mission of such a book as this is, of course, to discuss pregnancy, and, without being a textbook of obstetrics, it fulfills the mission very well. The medical-scientific information in this volume consists of the best current opinions. Ms. Gillis and Ms. Lichtendorf have taken pains to discuss the major matters relevant to pregnancy and to verify their facts with authoritative sources. Individual readers may find that they wish to review some of the statements made by the authors with their personal providers of care. Readers should also compare the information provided by many other sources with·the facts given in the book. This kind of patient education is highly desirable. The technically trained providers of health care, including obstetricians, nurse-midwives and nurse-practitioners, are educated to teach. They are, however, limited in the amount of time they can spend with individual patients in reviewing this body of information. Efforts are made to make up for this deficiency by group teaching, but there are clear limitations to this as well. The ideal is both individual and group instruction, supplemented by a competent source book such as this.

Of course, there continue to be controversies in obstetrics as in every other discipline in medicine. An incomplete understanding of these can give rise to anxiety. Patients may read or hear what purport to be authoritative presentations, and are then given what seem to be diametrically opposite opinions from their obstetricians. The authors have skillfully dealt with many of these issues and have succeeded in doing this in a reassuring, supportive and informative way.

There is simply no question that better-educated patients who participate in their own care do, in fact, have better outcomes. This not only is true in the completion of a normal process like pregnancy, but also has been observed repeatedly in the care of people with major illnesses, such as heart attacks, high blood pressure, diabetes, and even in the curability of malignancies. The basic message is educated consumerism.

There is also a good deal more to being pregnant than the medical data, however important the latter may be. It is in this area that this book may be of its greatest value. It goes into a number of areas that are not ordinarily deemed the concern of health care providers and about which they may not be fully informed. This includes such matters as the legal rights of pregnant women, availability of disability insurance, job safety and workers' compensation, and related social issues. This book provides

an important resource for information in these areas. It is
a reference work with which the reader can fill in the
gaps that may have been left by explanations that are
inadvertently too brief or too technical.

It is significant that Ms. Gillis and Ms. Lichtendorf
encourage the pregnant woman to be an active partici-
pant in her own care. There are difficulties inherent in
this, as we all recognize. The health care provider is a
trained professional equipped with a large body of technical information, and the patient is an amateur. This is
true in all doctor-patient relationships, and has the necessary result that the relationship is an unequal one. Further, all people seeking health care, even for a healthy
pregnancy, are dealing with a life crisis, which of necessity generates anxiety. The outcome of events cannot be
known, and all patients grasp the unpredictability of the
situation. These factors combine to create dependency
needs. In response to these needs the health care provider is cast in a parental role in relationship to the
patient, which itself may create problems.

Another factor of major importance in the United States
is that more than 90 percent of obstetricians are men. In
my conversations with the editor who has worked on this
book it has struck me that she consistently referred to the
obstetrician as *he.* Many of us responsible for training
physicians in this specialty have determined to train a
maximum number of women. However, the proportion of
women in medical schools in the United States at the
present time is approximately 30 percent, and only a
fraction of them enter obstetrics. The fraction is increasing, but it will be a few decades before any sizable
proportion of people providing obstetrical care is of women.
Perhaps one of the reasons for the growing popularity of
care by nurse-midwives is the fact that the overwhelming
majority of certified nurse-midwives in the United States
are women. Entry into the nursing profession has itself
been an expression of sexism in our society. It is certainly
not difficult to recognize that many women feel that they
can accomplish a basis of equality with another woman
more readily than they can with a man. An inequality of
relationships, which may not, in fact, be what any of the
participants actually want, is a hindrance to the provision

of health care. The sooner we can together reduce it, the better.

Well, again, what is new about pregnancy? Despite the success of the test-tube baby, women will continue to carry the fertilized egg to term over a period of some 265 days. Despite what is likely to be a transitory increase in the proportion of cesarean births, labor has not changed. What is new is the recognition that having a baby is wholly compatible with a woman's entire social and professional life. She can remain a fully realized person— and there can be nothing better for those who love her, particularly her child. Ms. Gillis and Ms. Lichtendorf, by writing this book, have made it easier for women to achieve this goal.

PREFACE

AN END TO
MATERNITY EXILE

This is a wonderful time to be pregnant. You can work—right up until labor and delivery if you like. You can participate in your medical care. You can live the type of pregnancy that is right for you now—not the type that was right for others years ago.

Today's pregnancy is an old game but with new rules. Although *you* may be living your nine months according to the new guidelines, you may be surprised to find out that many of those around you—your boss, your health care team, perhaps your husband or mother—may not yet have learned the new rules.

Pregnancy is not the end of you as a person. Childbearing is an accomplishment, but it will not be your only achievement. It is up to you to take charge of your pregnancy rather than to allow your pregnancy to take charge of you. In this book we plan to tell you how.

The Transition Has Already Begun

The New Pregnancy reflects the changes that in recent years have affected the social and economic status of women. There has been an enormous increase of women in the labor force; women are better educated, and the women's movement has encouraged us to look at ourselves and our lives differently. Accessible birth-control measures have made it possible for us to plan our families, and economic fluctuations are making the two-income family necessary to afford the essentials of life.

How do you fit into this scheme? For one thing, only a few years ago pregnancy meant a retreat from the world and a withdrawal from regular activities. Today pregnancy means continuing your normal life—albeit with a slightly more defined figure. Being pregnant is a terrific experience, but it no longer has to be a separate part of your life. It is an integral *part* of your life.

What else could be different about pregnancy today? Everything!

- At least 1.5 million pregnant women are in the work force today. Only a few years ago a woman was forced to leave her job when she became pregnant or started to "show." Your childbearing function can no longer serve as an excuse to limit your career opportunities.

- You have more legal protection than ever before because many forms of pregnancy-based discrimination are forbidden by law.

- You have more choices in the type of health care you can use during pregnancy and childbirth, and as a consumer of medical services, you can make more demands in the type of service you receive.

- Your family can participate in your pregnancy as never before.

- You can travel, continue your physical activities, and enjoy an active sex life.

- Most of all, you can live the active type of life you are used to living. You do not have to give it up simply because you are pregnant. Nevertheless, there may be those who think you should. It is to confront these outdated attitudes and old myths that we have written this book.

A Sharing of Experiences

In order to determine just what is happening today, we decided to talk with pregnant women across the country. After all, who knows more about the reality of being pregnant in America today? We wanted to know if women were really living a new type of pregnancy—or if the attitudes of those around them were preventing them from doing so. If barriers to an active pregnancy did exist, what, then, were these women doing to help eliminate them? We got our answers—and our aim is to pass them along to you.

In order to reach a wide dispersion of pregnant women, we placed advertisements and letters to the editor in a variety of publications. We invited pregnant women to share their experiences—good and bad—about such matters as working during pregnancy, physician relationships, legal problems, relationships with loved ones, everything relating to today's pregnancy.

Almost immediately, several hundred letters arrived. We were astonished at the response. Ultimately, we interviewed some two hundred pregnant women, either in person or by telephone.

We weren't attempting a scientific study. We were simply striving to determine *how* pregnant women lead their lives today in order to provide guidelines for you and the pregnant women of tomorrow.

We spoke with pregnant nurses, doctors, lawyers, factory workers, saleswomen, real estate brokers, travel agents, librarians, actresses, flight attendants, secretaries, newscasters, college professors and elementary school teachers. We spoke with women making $50,000 a year and with unsalaried homemakers. We spoke with women in their early twenties having their first babies, and with women having their first babies at forty; with women having a first baby in a second marriage, or a third child while working. These women expressed the spirit of the New Pregnancy—a freedom to be active and in charge of one's life.

We quickly learned that some women had better pregnancies than others—not necessarily because they were smarter or richer, but because they learned how to successfully manage their nine special months. It is their accumulated know-how, plus some substantial input from experts in many fields—geneticists, obstetricians, lawyers, psychologists, sports experts, travel agents, sex therapists—that we intend to pass along to you.

We also spoke with almost one hundred employers, both on and off the record, to learn how they looked at their pregnant employees. While pregnant women have been learning that they can work and be active, industry, union leaders, the medical profession and even the courts have not always recognized that a working pregnancy is both possible and desirable. For some people this has been a rude awakening.

The response from business was as encouraging as the response from the women themselves. In virtually every instance, companies were willing to share their experiences, and in turn wanted to know what other employers were doing regarding work conditions and benefit provisions for the growing number of pregnant employees. The information they shared with us will help you manage your pregnancy to your advantage and to your employer's satisfaction.

As a working pregnant woman in the late twentieth century, you will be concerned with new issues, such as the impact of an industrial environment on a developing baby; whether it is safe for a pregnant woman to work in a chemical plant; whether it is possible to detect genetic problems before birth. At work you are protected by legal rulings, but often these are unevenly applied. Pregnant women can be treated fairly by employers, but not all are. We will tell you how to recognize pregnancy-based discrimination and where to go for recourse. You have the right to the best medical care during your pregnancy, and we will try to help you find it. We will discuss obstetrical controversies, and we will tell you how to deal with doctors. Because women often have trouble in dealing with doctors, we will show you how to be treated as a whole person rather than a pelvis. We will give you information about nutrition, sex, alcohol, and how to balance pregnancy demands with your active way of living.

Women today have discovered the fun and challenge of physical activity and sports. Pregnancy is no reason to give them up. Though your doctor will give you the go-ahead, it is the sports-woman who's been pregnant who has the know-how. Therefore, we have gone to the top female pros who have had babies to learn what they did during their pregnancies to keep their games going right.

We will tell you how to see the outside world—how to fly to Europe, sail on a cruise ship and even be a tourist in the Middle East. And we will help you find out what is going on inside of you—not in your womb but in your inner self. Pregnancy is a time of many emotions, of ups and downs, fears and exhilaration.

As for sex, there is potential for great pleasure in pregnancy. We will set aside taboo and look at some of the medical facts. Then we'll discuss ways to keep alive sexually while pregnant and after the baby is born.

In the immediate past, if a woman became pregnant, she knew that she would spend years raising a child. Today, a woman often gives birth, returns to work after a short maternity leave and then finds herself tackling the difficult role of career person/mother. If a woman decides on motherhood as her career, her choice exposes her to other stress, because there are people who feel that motherhood is no longer the be-all and end-all. Therefore, although our major emphasis will be on the nine months of pregnancy, we have also included a chapter on coping with the conflicts and demands of new motherhood.

We have left the path of traditional pregnancy books for good reason. You are pregnant at a time of strong social change for women. The concept of pregnancy that we are offering is new and different from that of the past. It is one that you won't read about in medical books on pregnancy. In fact, this is the first pregnancy book to say that you may need a lawyer as much as an obstetrician!

You may still find problems, but times are changing. If you know what you are doing, know what to demand, know how to maneuver to get what you want, and anticipate the arguments you'll hear, you have a good chance of achieving your aims for the kind of pregnancy you want to have.

The women interviewed for this book have proven that an exciting, challenging pregnancy is entirely possible. So have the book's authors. One of us is a medical science writer who worked throughout her pregnancy and traveled extensively. The other is a corporate executive who not only conducted business here and overseas, but even landed a new and better job during her ninth month of pregnancy!

We have lived the New Pregnancy. It is with enthusiasm that we suggest that you try it.

THE NEW
PREGNANCY

1

AT WORK

Pregnancy alone can no longer shape or shorten your career path, since there are vast numbers of women now in the labor force—many of them in the prime childbearing years.

Look around your office, school or work place. Chances are there will be more than one contoured belly, as many of your coworkers have chosen to exercise the option of motherhood along with you. Although some eyebrows may still be raised at the sight of a swollen belly at work, it is becoming increasingly common for the working woman of today to remain on the job throughout her pregnancy and to return to her job shortly thereafter.

You may encounter some problems, but you will find your working pregnancy a new and exciting career challenge, one that can be handled with success, aplomb and visible results. Your pregnancy can be an exciting and wonderful experience, but you must recognize that

- For many women pregnancy is a career crisis.

- Society is only beginning to deal with women who work during pregnancy and who return to work afterwards.

- Employers have special concerns—and prejudices.

- There are important new laws that benefit working pregnant women, but they are unevenly applied and a company's individual policies may be more important in your particular case.

1

- In the eyes of the law and your employer your pregnancy does not dictate special treatment or sick leave.

- A woman's own attitude has a great deal to do with how she fares—confidence is contagious.

We plan to tell you just what rights you have as a pregnant employee, how to reassure your boss and associates that you are committed to your job and how best to manage successfully your nine months at work.

SETTING YOUR PRIORITIES: WHAT DO YOU WANT TO DO?

As soon as you confirm your pregnancy you should evaluate realistically your future plans. What exactly do *you* want to do? Do you want to work through your pregnancy, take a short maternity leave and immediately return to your job? Would you rather take an extended leave in order to spend a little more time at home with the baby? Would you rather stop work altogether? Do you want to use this time to relax and think about a change in career?

Be honest. If you are unsure about what you want to do, think about your options, write them down and try to determine what is important to you.

If you want to spend the early years with your child, you don't have to do much planning. If you intend to return to work after childbirth, the most important consideration is child care, since this is probably the major question that will arise when you are discussing your plans with your employer. Your employer is not prying. He wants to know how you are planning to care for the child so that he will be able to continue to depend upon you as an employee. It is a valid question. And you must feel that your baby is in good hands so that you will be able to concentrate on fulfilling the requirements of your job rather than on worrying about the child.

This is not too early to begin thinking about child care. In fact, the earlier you begin the process of determining what type of child care you want, the more satisfied you will be when you finally find it.

If you wait until your ninth month or until after you

come home from the hospital, you may have to settle for whatever is available. You may be dissatisfied; then what do you do? How do you explain this to your employer? Be practical and plan ahead.

Make a list of what's important to you with regard to child care. Ask your working friends what they think. Do you want one person to take care of your baby in your home? Are you willing to take your baby out of the house to another person's home or to a child-care center? What facilities are available in your area? What is the going rate for the different types of facilities in your area? And what are you willing to pay? Is the amount you must pay for child care more than you make?

Investigate the Internal Revenue Service stipulations for deduction of child-care costs. At present the government does not consider child care a truly deductible expense, and it allows only a limited form of tax credit. This is largely because a working wife's salary is still thought of as supplementary income. In general, 20 percent of approved child-care expenses for one child, up to a limit of $2,000, is deductible. This means that you may deduct $400 per child, maximum two children, from your taxes for child-care expenses. Thus, in all probability you will have to pay for your child-care expenses with after-tax dollars—or straight out of the money you earn.

How will you transport your child to your child-care facilities? Will your husband help with the chauffeuring? Is the age of your caretaker important to you as far as child-care arrangements are concerned? If you have someone come to your house, will your caretaker be expected to do any other chores? Must that person have her own transportation?

There are many more options for child care than you might normally think. Widows, women with grown children, university students, mates of students—there is a variety of sources in every community. Be creative. Ask around. Advertise. Interview and *check references*. Do not settle for second best. Start early and make sure you are completely comfortable with your child-care arrangements. This is one of the most important decisions you will make during this time.

How Difficult Is a Working Pregnancy?

It is important that you assess your weekly schedule and recognize that a working pregnancy may require a slight modification in your normal routine. Almost every pregnant woman suffers from feeling tired, even though she feels well. It is a normal part of any pregnancy, particularly in the first and last trimesters, because of the physical impact on the body. If you work, you owe it to your employer to be well rested and physically able to do your job. Since the days of superwoman are fading fast, you can feel free to pare down your activities in order to be most efficient on the job and at home. As one public-relations woman said, "When I was pregnant, I went to work every day. I did everything. I thought I was terrific. But my husband's reaction was, 'Sure, you were terrific in the office, but when you came home at night you were a wet rag.'"

- Make a list of your plans for the week, review them, and reschedule or eliminate some of the nonessential activities if you find yourself overbooked or overcommitted.

- Avoid schedule juggling or scheduling yourself down to the last minute. This builds up not only fatigue but anger as well.

- Concentrate on your work during the day, rest at night and limit your weekend entertainment.

- Divide the household responsibilities with your husband and stick to them. Do your half. If he doesn't complete his chores, then either leave them undone or hire someone to do them.

Once the bases have been covered, it is up to you to keep the nine months running smoothly. It is your responsibility to present an appropriate picture of yourself, not only for your own future with your employer, but for those pregnant women who will follow behind you.

Be Confident

Remember, you do not have to justify your pregnancy to anyone. You will not be a "bad" mother if you continue to work after the baby arrives, nor will you "cop out" if you choose to devote your time to the very serious and oftentimes difficult job of taking care of an infant.

Remember, too, that the pregnant working woman hasn't been around very long, so it is up to you to set the pace and to convey a positive attitude. You should also be aware that pregnancy does not entitle you to special treatment, and you should therefore minimize the importance of your pregnancy as far as your job is concerned.

Let's take the example of Sharon Hunt, who coaches and teaches swimming to children. Initially she was afraid to tell her boss about her pregnancy, because she was worried about his reaction and the reactions of the mothers of her young students. She was right in her assessment of both reactions. Her boss wanted her to leave "for safety's sake," and the mothers objected to her coaching their children. Sharon persisted because she felt she could do the job, although she agreed to work with a backup coach who could cover for her if she couldn't make the numerous meets. "It was early summer and I had morning sickness all the time, but I just worked around it. People were shocked at the beginning, but that didn't bother me, because I never considered stopping my regular activities. No one thought I'd make it through the nine months, but my husband is a student, so I had to keep working. We needed the money. Now the baby is almost due, and my boss is telling me that I really taught him something. He's even conceded that I did a good job—and the mothers are looking at me differently too."

Assess the Medical Fact of Your Working Pregnancy

Whether it is safe and healthy for pregnant women to work is a current topic of considerable discussion. The question of health largely relates to the physical and emotional aspects of pregnancy; the question of safety, to occupational hazards.

Because the safety of the pregnant woman in the work force has become a political and social issue pitting women's groups, labor unions, and safety and health agencies against industry, it is important for you to know what you can do to best assess your *own* medical situation. Although the term "occupational hazard" is most often considered as a condition of industrial work, there are a variety of work situations that can be hazardous to the pregnant woman in any normal office environment. For instance, a secretary who sits too long in one position could get varicose veins or leg cramps.

Occupational Hazards and the Pregnant Woman: A New Problem

In the 1960's federal equal-employment legislation opened the doors of a variety of new work places for women, and researchers began to look at industrial substances that appeared to affect development of the fetus—for instance, lead, vinyl chloride and radiation (which may also cause sperm abnormalities in men). It became apparent that some medical guidance was needed. However, it wasn't until 1976 that the National Institute for Occupational Safety and Health funded a study group and contracted with the American College of Obstetricians and Gynecologists to look at this problem. The result was a 72-page document entitled *Guidelines on Pregnancy and Work*. It is important to you because it is currently the only broad-based statement on whether it is safe to work during pregnancy. It states that it *is* safe for you to work, depending upon you, the state of your health, the kind of pregnancy you are having, and how and where you work. A 1980 ACOG technical bulletin, "Pregnancy, Work and Disability," further expanded these guidelines and stated that "with infrequent exceptions . . . the normal woman with an uncomplicated pregnancy and a normal fetus in a job that presents no greater potential hazards than those encountered in normal daily life in the community may continue to work without interruption until the onset of labor and may resume working several weeks after an uncomplicated delivery." In other words, the pregnant woman as an active and important part of the work force has received "official" recognition. We have printed an excerpt of these guidelines on pages 221–23 to give you the means to assess your own medical and work situation with your physician or health support team so you can make a joint decision about the safety of your work during pregnancy.

To provide good obstetrical care under the NIOSH–ACOG guidelines, a physician is supposed to record a work history at the first prenatal visit, and update and review it at subsequent visits. It may actually be taken by a nurse or physician's assistant, or may be a form to be completed by the woman herself. This history is very important, because physicians may have to be educated about what it means for a woman to work.

If you are concerned about occupational hazards, it is especially important that *you* take the initiative and discuss your medical concerns about your job, first with your physician and then, if necessary, with your employer. Follow the guideline form (pages 221–23), and discuss each set of questions with your physician or health support team. Be as honest and complete as possible. Keep in mind that pregnancy is a dynamic situation and that modifications in your job duties—which should be discussed jointly with your own physician and your company's occupational health specialist—may not only be better for your health, but may help you continue to be a productive employee. Many physicians, for instance, will suggest modifications that allow a patient to continue working, if not at your regular job, then at another task. Tell him exactly what you do, what your hours are, whether you have slack time and rest periods, what the pace is. Describe your working environment, everything from the accessibility of clean bathrooms to the noise level, amount of vibration and airborne dusts at work, and, of course, specific chemicals you are in contact with. If you do not know what they are, ask your employer what hazardous substances you may have been exposed to. You have a right to this information. For some women, such as carpenters, waitresses and laundry workers, physical work is an obvious hazard. For others the danger is subtle, as, for example, for office workers or salespeople who must do prolonged sitting or standing. Women who must lift or pull heavy loads should discuss their tasks.

It is also important that your physician be aware of the type of work you do because it may affect the point at which you cease working toward the end of your pregnancy. For instance, those women who perform more strenuous jobs may be required to stop work six weeks prior to delivery, those who do a moderate amount of bending, stooping, lifting or twisting, four weeks before delivery and those who perform office or clerical tasks, two weeks before delivery.

There are no guidelines for the homemaker, but it is important to discuss the conditions of this work place as well. This means talking about household chemicals, sprays, paints, cleaning and gardening materials, about carrying a load of groceries *and* a toddler while pregnant with another child. If ladder climbing is considered hazardous for pregnant women in industry (which it often is because of a change in balance and a tendency to get dizzy), it can be just as hazardous for the woman at home.

Is It Safe for You to Work?

Once a physician has obtained a realistic work history and has assessed your obstetrical health profile, he or she can make a recommendation. If there is no "excessive" exposure to threatening elements (for example, chemicals), if you are in good health or if you have a condition that can be controlled medically, you can usually continue working. In some cases a physician may suggest modifications. In all recommendations about work during pregnancy, it is important to ask how long they are to be in force. There are a series of physiological changes during pregnancy. The nausea that may have caused a pregnant woman difficulty on her job early in pregnancy and that may be a reason for a work adjustment may be no problem later in pregnancy.

There are some women who are advised *not* to work during pregnancy, as, for example, the woman who has or develops a severe, threatening obstetrical or health condition, or the woman who is exposed to excessive risk at a work place where modifications or transfers to safety can't be achieved.

You should be aware that some of the changes of pregnancy can make you more susceptible to work or environmental influences. For example, anemia is common in pregnancy and may be compounded by substances such as carbon monoxide and lead. During pregnancy, because of the baby's oxygen demands and changes in your own breathing system, you can suffer from chemicals in the air in amounts that are "allowable" for nonpregnant workers. Although no worker should have to perform in conditions where the floor is slippery—and many women in industrial labor report that they do—this is not advised for pregnant women at all.

Before worrying, you should look at the chart of typical work exposures on pages 224–27. Then, if you have questions, you should speak with your physician or a local office of the National Institute for Occupational Safety and Health (pages 227–29). You can also turn to the university medical school nearest you that has a department of obstetrics and occupational medicine or the equivalent (pages 237–38).

UNDERSTANDING YOUR LEGAL RIGHTS AND ECONOMIC BENEFITS

After you have assessed your medical situation, you must determine two additional factors: What are your employer's economic policies, that is, what about health insurance coverage, temporary disability payments during your absence or your employer's general leave policy; and what is your employer's attitude—is he or she prejudiced?

Now ask yourself

- What type of employer do I work for? Is it a large corporation with set policies or a small company with informal rules? If it is a large corporation with set policies, it will be easier to determine *exactly* to what you are entitled.

- How long have I been with the company? If you are a long-term employee with a proven track record, you will probably have an easier time than a newly employed person.

- Where am I in the office pecking order? If you are in a position that is tailored to a particular skill or has been developed through your own personal capabilities, your employer *may* be more willing to make an effort to accommodate your pregnancy and future plans than if you are in an easily replaceable position.

Once you have determined what *type* of employer you work for and where you stand in the organization, you should then begin to determine your rights as a pregnant woman in your company.

Your Legal Rights As a Pregnant Employee

As a pregnant woman today you *do* have certain legal rights—but the *extent* of these rights largely depends on your employer.

There are three basic areas of concern regarding your rights as a pregnant woman. The first deals with job discrimination and is comprised of issues with which most people are familiar. It covers such topics as discrimination in hiring, firing, promotions, job security and mandatory leave policies—the type of employment practices that we normally associate with inequitable treatment.

The second area involves money—and primarily relates to your benefits during pregnancy. There are two basic types of benefits: (1) medical coverage for your pregnancy, labor and delivery, and (2) employer or state benefits covering the period of time when you stop working to have your baby to the time when you return to your job. If you do not return to your job, you are not entitled to these leave benefits.

The third issue is occupational health and safety. This is a completely new area, and it is marked by a variety of concerns. For our purposes it applies to employers who refuse to hire women of childbearing age because of potential exposure to toxic substances, or who transfer pregnant women to positions that are usually safer but lower paying. This is an area in flux, with few hard and fast decisions having been made at this point.

A Major Breakthrough: What the Law Says

Pregnant women *do* have rights—and a 1978 law, The Pregnancy Discrimination Act (P.L. 95–555) passed by the U.S. Congress now specifically provides for protection against pregnancy-based discrimination. The law, which amends Title VII of the 1964 Civil Rights Act, specifically prohibits employment discrimination based on pregnancy, childbirth or related medical conditions. Title VII of the 1964 Civil Rights Act, as you may be aware, has been the most effective tool to date for dealing with sex discrimination, and has been widely used by the Equal Employment Opportunity Commission (the federal agency responsible for enforcing this law) to stop employers from discriminatory practices.

You are very lucky to be a working pregnant woman now, because the unfair 1976 ruling, *General Electric* v. *Gilbert*, in which the U.S. Supreme Court found that bias against pregnant workers in employee health insurance plans was *not* sex discrimination, has now been superseded by the amendment to Title VII.

The bypass bill means that you are not only covered against pregnancy-based discrimination in such areas as hiring, firing, seniority, promotion, job security and mandatory leave policies, you are also covered by any temporary disability or sick leave plan your employer may have.

Although the new law bars discrimination based on pregnancy, it does *not* require employers to grant pregnant employees preferential treatment in hiring, continued employment, or coverage under sick leave, health or disability plans. In addition, employers are *not* required to establish *new* benefit programs if none exist.

TYPES OF MATERNITY PROVISIONS

Most employers offer some sort of group health insurance, and at least some portion of maternity medical costs is usually covered. Some plans may be better than others, so it doesn't hurt to check your own situation.

Many pregnant women assume that because their group health policy covers maternity, every pregnancy-related bill is covered by their health insurance. This is often not the case. Make sure you know what your policy covers. (See the insurance checklist on page 13.)

In order to avoid conflicts and misunderstandings about your pregnancy-related costs, it is essential to know what your own company policy is and what your benefits are concerning coverage and maternity leave. In general, most employers fall into the following categories:

- *Those who pay for leaves of absence*. This employer treats pregnancy as any other disability, and covers the employee's full or partial salary and benefits from the time she is away from the office until after the birth of the baby.

- *Those who partially pay for leaves of absence*. This employer provides for partial disability pay and/or unpaid leave of absence. Benefits are also usually continued during absence.

- *Those who do not pay for leaves of absence*. This employer does not provide for pregnancy disability pay. However, an unpaid leave of absence is usually granted, and benefits usually continue. You may be covered by state pregnancy disability coverage provisions. In some cases, the employer does not provide maternity coverage, nor does the state.

There are two specific types of employee benefits relating to pregnancy. Medical insurance is usually provided for most workers through some sort of group health plan, and it pays for all or a portion of your medical care and related medical services. The other kind of benefit, as we've already discussed, is temporary disability coverage, which provides for paid "leave" time, or that portion of time when you are away from your job due to some temporary physical condition.

Medical Insurance

Having a baby is expensive, with costs varying widely from state to state and locality to locality. If you recognize this and plan accordingly, you won't be hit with any major surprises when the baby arrives. Some health plans pay for full coverage, others pay for partial coverage, and others include coverage only as an option in their medical insurance program.

There are also new types of health delivery systems—specifically, health maintenance organizations (HMOs)—in which you pay a monthly fee covering health and hospital care and in turn receive such services as maternity care paid in full.

Most employers have a written guide concerning

insurance and other benefits, so read it until you thoroughly understand what your plan will pay for during your pregnancy, labor and delivery. If you are uncertain about what your health plan provides, ask your personnel or benefits officer to explain it to you.

Questions to Ask about Your Medical Insurance

● What is the type and extent of coverage that you have? The amount of medical insurance you have may depend on your salary level.

● What does your health insurance cover? Doctor or health support team bills? Office visits? Delivery costs? Hospital stay?

● Is it full or partial coverage? Must you use a specific medical service (you might if you use an HMO), or are you able to choose your own?

● Does it cover any medication you may require during or after delivery? Does it cover complications or cesarean section? (If so, is it full or partial coverage? This may be important, because the cost for cesarean section is about double that of a normal delivery.)

● Does it cover hospital nursery costs or any special infant care that may be required in the hospital?

● Does the plan stipulate that you pay the bills directly to the receiver and the insurance then reimburses you? Or does your plan provide that the insurance pays the hospital and health team directly?

● When does insurance coverage for the baby begin? Is it at birth or when you come home from the hospital? Be sure to notify your insurance carrier to put your baby on your policy as a dependent.

● Does your hospital require that you pay any costs your insurance does not cover before they will discharge you?

You should also discuss the effect of your maternity leave on seniority, career advancement, regular merit increases, pension and retirement plan contributions, and vacation accruals.

How to Double-Check Your Company's Medical Insurance

One thing you might check out discreetly if your company does not provide maternity coverage is whether the wives of male employees receive medical insurance coverage for maternity costs. If they do, you may well have grounds for a discrimination claim. You must check around first, however, to find out whether your employer is arbitrarily discriminating in the type of health insurance he is providing to employees, or whether this is permissible under your state insurance code.

Many state insurance commissions have regulations that mandate what *must* be included in policies sold to employers in a particular state. In some instances maternity coverage may be required; in others it may be what is termed a "permissible policy exclusion" under an employer's health insurance plan, and may *not* be required.

If you feel you are not being fairly treated, call your state insurance commissioner and find out what the requirements of your state are with regard to insurance policies and maternity coverage. (See the listings on pages 237–44 for locations and telephone numbers.) Most state insurance commissions have minimum regulations stating what an insurance company must offer in its policies. Ask what must be included regarding maternity coverage in insurance policies sold in your state, and then compare this with what your *own* policy provides.

Many state insurance commissions have consumer affairs departments, and some have toll-free numbers. Most are located in the state capital, but many have regional offices. They are there to serve you as the consumer, so feel free to ask questions.

You may also want to call the insurance company that has written your policy to ask what they provide in maternity coverage. Use the checklist on page 13 as a guideline to determine what questions to ask. Then compare it with what your employer provides and what the state insurance commission requires. If the provisions do not match up, you may have grounds for a complaint.

Whenever you talk with the insurance carrier, make sure that you write down the name of the person with whom you speak, the dates and a summary of your conversation. It may be useful if you have to file a discrimination claim.

If you feel that you are receiving unfair treatment, then ask your benefits officer or supervisor for a written statement of exactly to what you are entitled, and an explanation of why this is inconsistent with the coverage provided for other medical conditions, with that provided for the wives of male employees, or with the state insurance requirements.

If you get an unsatisfactory answer and want to fight it, then file a complaint through the appropriate in-house procedures, and if this fails, through the appropriate state agency. (See pages 245–49 in the appendix for how to file a complaint.)

The Other Kind of Coverage—Temporary Physical Disability Coverage

The law states that if your employer provides temporary disability coverage for other temporary physical disabilities, then he must also provide it for yours. If your employer does *not* provide temporary disability coverage for any employee, then he does not have to provide it for you just because you are pregnant.

Temporary disability provisions cover only that period of time when you are unable to work. This usually is from slightly before to immediately after childbirth or at some point during your pregnancy if your health support team indicates that complications prevent you from working.

A leading feminist lawyer, active in women's rights legislation, explained maternity leave this way: "Maternity leave does not mean that you can take a month off to fix up the kiddie's room. Nor is it leave to take care of the kiddies. Maternity leave is that period of time when Mom is away from her job, when she is recuperating from childbirth, is disabled and is unable to work."

Still Other Benefits—From Your State

If your employer does not have a temporary disability plan, then you may be eligible for all or partial unemployment or temporary disability benefits from your state. Not all states provide coverage, and it differs from state to state. Once again, it covers only that period of time when you are away from your job and unable to work. If your state does not provide for temporary disability coverage for maternity and your employer does not have a plan to cover temporary disabilities, then you are not eligible for any benefits.

Make sure you know what your state provides if you are not covered by your employer. The state agencies that normally cover these provisions are listed on pages 254–60. Because state regulations can and do change frequently, however, you must check with your own state to determine the current regulations and whether they might apply to you.

State payments, which will probably be a portion of your weekly salary, are intended to provide basic financial support during that period of time when you are unable to work. They are not a gift from the state.

There may be a waiting time after you file your claim before your benefits arrive, so ask the agency when you can expect to receive your money and whether it will be paid weekly or in one lump sum at the end of your disability period. Ask for the name of the person handling your file, so that if you need to follow up you'll know whom to call. And make copies of everything that you can. Bureaucracies sometimes lose track of papers!

If your physician has to sign forms, send them to him or her with a self-addressed, stamped envelope and a note explaining what they are. Request that he or she process them as soon as they are received. Follow this up with a phone call in three days and another if need be. Your employer may also have to sign a similar form stating that you are employed, that you will be returning to work and that he does not provide for temporary disability coverage.

If you have not heard anything within a week or two after filing, call and ask what the status of your claim is. Most agencies will send you a notice stating that your claim has been either accepted or rejected. If your claim has been rejected, call and ask why. Then ask for a written explanation. If you are rejected, you may want to file an appeal. If this is the case, ask what the procedure is and follow the appropriate format.

ASSESSING YOUR EMPLOYMENT SITUATION—STRATEGICALLY

Although many women do work successfully through their pregnancies, others experience resistance or outright hostility from their employers. In order for you to have the best possible working pregnancy, you must look at yourself through your employer's eyes, position yourself so that you are sensitive to your employer's needs and interests, and carry through accordingly with your plans for coping with these potentially hostile reactions. You know you are an important and serious part of the work force, but your employer has certain worries about pregnant employees as they relate to him or her and to the job.

The Concerns of Employers

Your pregnancy is an inconvenience. Questions running through your employer's mind include, How long will she be out? What will I have to do during her absence? What problems will this create for me? Will I have to hire someone—even temporarily—to replace her? Will I have to spend time training someone to cover for her? What about my vacation?

Consider that even if a colleague breaks a limb or has a heart attack and must be away from the office for an unspecified amount of time, the expectations for a woman—especially a pregnant one—are different. If the working pregnant woman is not a common occurrence in your office, school or place of work, then you must consider what effect your pregnancy is going to have, not only on your immediate superior but on his superior and beyond. In all likelihood your boss will have to defend you to the next level up in terms of promotion, salary, career advancement and so forth. So think of how your pregnancy will reflect upon your boss.

"If a woman is serious, knows she is upwardly mobile

and has a good relationship with her superior, I hope she would share her plans, just as if she was considering a move to another part of the country," said one employer. "If one of my employees saw me spinning cartwheels for her in the company in order to get her promoted, in the sense of fairness I hope she would keep me informed about her pregnancy. The pregnant career woman should look a little down the road and think of what her new boss might say to the person who promoted her—something like, 'Hey, John, did you know ahead of time that this woman was pregnant?' "

Here's an example of exactly this type of situation. A pregnant assistant manager of investor relations was being considered for a promotion. Though she was in the early stages of pregnancy, she discussed it with her boss, whose response was neither positive nor negative but rather, "What are *we* going to do about it, so that there are no negative effects through the company?"

She was given the promotion, but not until *after* she had the baby. Only then was she permitted to assume the responsibilities and receive the salary increase.

"It was called getting screwed," said the woman, "but I couldn't really do anything about it. I had to think of where I was in my career, the support I had in the company and the support my boss had. I lost about six months of higher pay, but sometimes in a time of transition it's better to consider strategy as a team rather than go it alone." She has since received two more promotions.

An administrative vice-president for a small New Jersey computer firm talked about the inconvenience of pregnancy: "When a woman breaks the news, her boss or employer is usually confronted with something that has never been discussed openly, because a woman doesn't want to say anything for fear of losing her job. By the time an employer hears about it, it is usually a fait accompli. The announcement is made at a time that is not a relaxing period for her, because she is usually on edge just about informing her employer. And he's probably busy and has little time to spend on discussing such things. When the news is broken it is usually not the most ideal situation anyway. We've had about fifteen pregnancies in the past three or four years, and I don't think I've ever heard anyone say, 'I'm planning to get pregnant in a few months—what about my job situation?' "

Although there are questions of personal freedom involved, here is an alternative you as a professional woman might consider: planning your pregnancy with your employer. As an executive of one of the world's largest multinational corporations said, "Professional women usually make their career plans ahead of time prior to becoming pregnant, and they carry these plans out. Pregnancy is just consistent with their career planning process. Although technically we're not able to talk about someone's pregnancy plans, it is probably of some significance to us to talk about it as a consideration in her career plans."

Although there have been many attempts to push aside the pregnancy issue, many employers are accepting pregnancy as just one more aspect of life in the labor force. With women comprising almost 50 percent of the labor force, they have little choice.

So while your pregnancy may be somewhat of an inconvenience for your employer, more often than not it will be accepted. It is up to you to make it a good experience.

You may possibly abuse company policy. Employers sometimes feel that women abuse privileges during and after pregnancy. One commonly expressed fear is that a pregnant woman will take excessive sick days. Another is that she will go on leave, be paid disability for her absence and then leave the company.

There are some women who will always take advantage of a situation, just as their male colleagues might, but in general pregnant women do not deliberately abuse sick leave. Most pregnant women who say that they want to work are serious about their intentions. Make sure you tell your employer what your plans are and then stick with them. Your employer will respond better to you and to those who follow you if you are fair in your expectations of yourself and of him.

Your pregnancy is an added cost to the company. Though there is evidence that attitudes are beginning to shift—that inconvenience can be handled and abuse of company policies can be limited—your employer still has one major concern about your pregnancy and its relation to him—economics. Cost to the employer is the bottom line of the controversy over fair and equal treatment of pregnancy-related disability coverage in this country, because it affects budgets, the planning process and, ultimately, the profitability of a company. Although other attitudes can be countered with valid arguments, the dollars-and-cents consideration is more difficult to confront.

These additional costs include health-insurance plans (which fully or partially cover maternity costs), temporary disability payments while the employee is on maternity leave, retraining or opportunity costs to hire and retrain a new employee if the pregnant woman leaves her job permanently, and costs for a replacement for the pregnant woman while she is away from her job after the baby is born. These are real costs, and it is justifiable for an employer to express concern over them.

Nevertheless, if employers want to recruit and retain good employees, then pregnancy-related costs should be regarded as a routine part of a company's health package, not as an outstanding "special" allocation.

As more women become aware of what is being done around the country with regard to pregnancy provisions (and many companies *do* offer outstanding benefit programs) and as the working pregnant woman becomes so common as to eliminate the concerns of employers, then the issues of inconvenience, abuse and cost will inevitably become less sensitive.

MANAGING YOUR WORKING PREGNANCY

How and When to Tell Your Employer about Your Pregnancy

Are you legally obligated to inform your employer of your pregnancy? No, but many *individual* companies require it as part of their general overall employment agreement.

If you are in a position to call your own shots, are extremely confident of your job situation and are in a stable industry where economic fluctuations will not affect your position, then you may want to consider not informing your superior. Pregnancy really *shouldn't* affect the way you handle your job.

If you do elect to inform your employer, make your announcement simple and direct. Tell your boss when you expect to deliver and how long you expect to work through your pregnancy. If you do *not* intend to return to work, then say so and offer to help train a replacement. But if you *do* plan to return to work, make sure that your employer knows that you do not plan for your pregnancy to interfere with your career goals.

Keep in mind, however, that no matter how much planning you do, no one knows—not even you—how you and your family are going to respond to that baby and how that baby is going to respond to you.

Here is an example of a well-structured pregnancy announcement: "I informed my superior first and laid out my plans for him in a very straightforward manner," a thirty-two-year-old marketing executive said. "During our discussion I said that I knew it was difficult to evaluate how much time I would be out with the child, but that my *intent* was to be out as short a period of time as possible—and to manage my job between the time I was out and the time I came back without being replaced."

Superiors take their cues from employees themselves, and your boss can also sense if you are being unrealistic. If you refuse to acknowledge potential problems and delays, and insist that nothing is going to be different—that you plan to deliver on Friday and to return to work on Monday—questions are apt to arise, because no one can be that sure of anything. When an employee begins to act this way, it is a clue that she has some real doubt in her mind, and employers respond accordingly. It makes them feel that perhaps the woman is unsure of herself. If you are uncertain about your plans, be open about your uncertainty. You can review your plans again toward the end of your pregnancy. Your employer will respect you more for your openness, and you will feel more comfortable about your plans. If you encounter resistance or outright discrimination, we will show you later in this chapter how to deal with it.

Put the news about your pregnancy in writing. This will give you documentation if you run into problems down the road and decide to file a pregnancy-based discrimination claim. Make sure you give a copy to your superior and to the personnel office. If you are not sure of your plans, say so in your note and offer to discuss them again at a later point in your pregnancy.

Break the news personally to your friends, assistants and subordinates, so they hear it from you rather than through the office grapevine.

To avoid charges that you are abusing company policy, make sure your job duties are covered, and arrange with your superior to have your responsibilities taken care of during your absence. In virtually every situation where other people are involved, this should be considered.

Do not expect others to respond favorably to you if it means more work for them. You will ensure less hostility and more enthusiasm if you tie up loose ends and assure others that you are not abandoning your work load. Do not let other members of the team down.

Although it may be a bit more work for you, help prepare those who will be covering for you by writing a series of notes and memos about your duties and related activities. Doing this shows your superiors and associates that you mean business. It also helps them to do your job your way, and it will save you the trouble of having to undo or re-do work when you return.

Arrange schedules in advance. If you must work a certain number of hours or have a revolving schedule that involves night and weekend work, make your schedule up early so that toward the end of your pregnancy you can work days only and get your rest at night. A brief memo to your superior stating that you have complied with these job requirements by fulfilling the night or weekend hours during the early part of your pregnancy will serve to inform him that *you* have met your obligations.

In cases you do tell your employer ahead of time and he or she doesn't provide for coverage of your duties until the last minute, your written notes will serve as proof that *you* were the cooperative party and cannot be faulted for your boss's failure to provide adequately for a smooth transition.

Try to wear appropriate clothing. Business dress is business dress, pregnant or not, and your image and appearance is particularly important at this time. (See more about this in Chapter Seven, "The Outer You.") How you come across visually may well affect how your company responds to you. So give careful consideration to your clothing and grooming.

Dealing with the Attitudes of Employers and Associates

Your superiors and associates may intentionally or unintentionally affect your emotional outlook at work and arouse unforeseen conflict or guilt. If you are being hassled, try to understand why. Then try to work out a solution.

A thirty-one-year-old lawyer informed her superior of her pregnancy as soon as she knew of it, writing her plans in a formal memo, stating that she hoped to maintain her level of activity during her pregnancy, have the baby and return to work after a few months. This is what happened to her: "I expected my office to be a lot more open-minded. I didn't foresee the hostile reaction. My boss told me that women were lawyers or mothers, but not both. There were a lot of hard feelings. My associates supported me, but management disagreed.

"I was determined to maintain my dignity and not shrink into the walls, but I knew I was being ignored. It was obvious that I wasn't receiving work. I stopped enjoying my job, because they made it so uncomfortable for me."

There is no set answer for dealing with every situation, but the most effective way to deal with such a negative attitude is to sit down with your boss and talk it out. You might say that it strikes you that his or her attitude is coming from within, and you would like to try to work it out. Would he or she please try to set aside personal prejudices and see this pregnancy as a part of you as a career person who happens to be female, of you as a future parent, and of you as a person who intends to work a long time at her job. See what the response is. Calmly answer any questions that may arise.

The way a company or institution treats you during your pregnancy may well be an indication of how they will treat you afterward. Even if you have the best of child-care arrangements and the most cooperative husband, you will inevitably have days after you return to work when you must stay home because of childhood illnesses, caretaker problems or other unforeseen events. Consider that how your firm reacts to you now is a sign of things to come.

If you have exhausted all possibilities for breaking down prejudices about your pregnancy and motherhood, you may ultimately have to leave your job. Trained women are desirable commodities today; if the job breaks down, don't be afraid to look for another.

One of the major reasons your associates may create problems is that they fear your pregnancy will mean more work for them. Their comments may come from nonacceptance rather than criticism. What can you do? If your pregnancy becomes a focus of conversation among your peers and if criticism or comments make you uncomfortable, let your critic have it—but with dignity.

Teachers have different problems from women who work in business and industry, since they deal primarily with students. At one time it was considered detrimental for students, especially in the elementary grades, to be aware of a teacher's pregnancy. Now educators view a teacher's pregnancy as educative. A New England superintendent of schools said, "Ten or fifteen years ago, some parents might have objected to a pregnant teacher, but now it's looked on as a learning experience. We get the children involved. It's just a part of life."

A woman who has worked for years to establish herself and has achieved respect in her field may suddenly discover that she is classified as a deserter by her feminist colleagues, both married and single.

A thirty-one-year-old Iowa district attorney told us: "For years I've been active in women's issues, ERA ratification, legal rights, and all of a sudden my female colleagues were telling me that I've copped out. I don't know whether I was hurt, angry or confused, but it was a completely unsettling experience."

The criticism may arise from your associates' own self-doubts or anxieties about how others might perceive them. Duke University historian William Chafe, author of *Women and Equality,* offered this explanation: "I think this is primarily a psychological reaction. Obviously, single women and career women who opt not to have children are threatened by women who choose to have a career and children, because this represents one more option that they have rejected or perhaps said couldn't be done." You must remember that by having a child you are upsetting the woman-as-either/or theory. Women colleagues can exhibit the same outdated or confused attitudes as your male colleagues, and expect that if you are going to compete on equal terms in a male world, then you cannot be a mother as well. If you sense a real prejudice and decide to confront your critics, consider the following questions:

- Who are these women and what is your relation to them?

- Is your relationship job-related? If so, what are your job requirements? Are they compromised by your pregnancy?

- Are you aware of any home, family or pregnancy-related conflicts or anxieties that these women might have?

- Do you value the friendships or associations enough to work it out?

- Are you secure in your own feelings about your pregnancy?

When you have considered these questions, if you decide to confront your critics you might want to consider the following points as a basis for your discussion:

- The criticism has nothing to do with your job.

- What is right for one person may not be right for another.

- Motherhood does not preclude a career.

Planning for Physical Contingencies

Even if you have done your best to consider your employer's concerns, have broken the news in a direct manner, have adequately provided for coverage during your ab-

sence and have carried yourself with confidence, you
may still encounter a variety of unexpected problems.

No matter how thoroughly you plan or how well you
feel at the beginning of your pregnancy, there is no way
to know what can happen as your pregnancy progresses.
Here are a few examples of physical contingencies and
how they were met.

- A thirty-seven-year-old advertising executive was confined to
  bed for most of the second half of her pregnancy. She continued her job by running a business telephone line into her
  house; her husband and secretary cooperated by running a
  courier service; and she was able to service her clients with
  the knowledge she had from years of experience on the job.

- Three weeks before her due date, a twenty-nine-year-old
  Kansas City engineer began to dilate. Her doctor gave her
  orders to spend a week in bed. Her office had not had much
  experience with engineers getting pregnant, but they treated
  her the same as anyone else would have been treated if he or
  she had been ill.

- Two weeks before her due date, a communications specialist
  was confined to bed with preeclampsia (a condition associated
  with high blood pressure, protein in the urine and unusual
  puffiness or swelling). She had just been finishing prepara-
  tions for her company's annual meeting, to be held within the
  next few days. She explained her condition to her superior,
  associates and assistant, and asked for their cooperation. Her
  staff came to her apartment to work out the final arrangements; she gave directions from her bedroom and the annual
  meeting went off smoothly.

- An Ann Arbor lawyer couldn't hold her urine, beginning with
  the seventh month of her pregnancy. She had a heavy trial
  schedule and wanted to complete her pending cases before
  she delivered. Wearing as many as three large sanitary nap-
  kins at a time, she went to court, changing as frequently as
  recesses permitted—and got her work done.

Arranging for Your Return

To explore the options for the postpregnancy period, talk
with your superior. Many companies now have flexible
"flexitime," or part-time work options, depending on the
job and the individual.

Keep a copy of any memos you write concerning your job. Among the things to keep a record of are the following:

- The announcement of your pregnancy to your superior and to personnel.

- A review of the plans you have made for your work to be covered and by whom.

- The benefits to which you are entitled.

- Notes of any time taken off for medical appointments or other absences, and copies of memos to your superior explaining your medical appointments and saying you expect to be away from _____ to _____. This can be useful if the subject of a raise is broached in succeeding months or if someone thinks you took too much time off during your pregnancy.

One final point. After you have your baby, your office will probably not know whether or not to contact you. You should make that decision. If you are planning to return but would like a few weeks alone with your new baby, then say so; if you would prefer to keep in touch with the office and show that you still feel responsible for projects that you have been involved in, check in every so often to touch base, and tell your colleagues to call you if anything comes up that they need to discuss with you.

Remember that you set the stage. If you consider your employer's needs, if you approach the nine months with a bit of practicality and planning, and if you pace yourself to get the most out of your physical capabilities, you will have a pregnancy that works successfully. If you *do* run into trouble, however, the next section will tell you how to cope with it.

PREPARING FOR POSSIBLE PROBLEMS

Now that you've thought through your personal options, learned about your employer's benefits and maternity policy, considered your boss's concerns, and have begun to manage your working pregnancy, you may think it will be smooth sailing. Possibly it will be. Then again, you may be surprised to discover that you are the recipient of

pregnancy-based discrimination although you have a terrific working relationship with your boss.

Even if you can recognize pregnancy-based discrimination, you may not have success with your employer regarding the possibility of changing company policies, or
you may not know how to go about this. Ultimately, you
may have to file a complaint with an outside agency.
There are three ways: through your union, if you are a
member, through your state, or through a federal civil-
rights agency.

Maternity discrimination takes several forms: refusal of
jobs to women who are or who *might* become pregnant;
unpaid pre- and/or post-childbirth maternity leaves; forced
resignations or outright discharges; inequitable medical or
disability benefits; loss of seniority and other accrued
benefits; and arbitrary employer policies regarding the
times and conditions for reemployment.

To determine whether or not you are being discriminated against on the basis of pregnancy, you should be
familiar with your employer's policies. In general, the
following principles should apply. They have been suggested by Ruth Weyand, a supervisory trial attorney on
the staff of the EEOC and the lawyer who argued the
landmark pregnancy disability case against General
Electric.

- If you are fully able to work, you should be treated the same
  as any other able-bodied worker.

- If you are partially disabled and your employer regularly
  assigns work to partially disabled employees, your employer
  should do the same for you.

- When you are temporarily unable to work due to childbirth or
  complications from pregnancy, your employer should give
  you the same rights to retain or accrue seniority, to accumulated sick pay and vacation credit, and to be paid sick pay,
  disability and health benefits, as any other employees who
  are temporarily disabled.

- You should have the costs of doctor and hospital bills for
  prenatal care, delivery and postnatal care paid by your employer without any more deductible or any further expenses

other than apply to doctor and hospital bills if your employer provides medical insurance benefits.

● You should be permitted to return to your job, just as other employees with temporary disability conditions.

The most important factor to consider is your ability to do your job. If you can function as you did before pregnancy, the fact that you are pregnant should have no bearing on your job.

Your employer may not be aware that his practices are discriminatory. Often, employers, as well as employees, don't consider sex discrimination to be a serious offense. Racial and religious discrimination is assumed to be far more serious.

Many employers, though, *are* aware of the law and have chosen to disregard or flout it. It may be because of the added expense in eliminating discriminatory practices. It may be because the employer does not believe a pregnant woman to be a serious employee. Or it may be because no one has challenged company policies.

Once again, what you must look for is clear-cut evidence that pregnancy is not treated by your employer on an equal basis with other temporary disabilities. These policies are not always written in a book, so you may have to do a little discreet investigation. It is important to ask around, get as much from the grapevine as possible and find out what has been granted to others with temporary physical disabilities. If you know of someone who has been granted extended leave for a disability, such as a broken limb from a skiing accident or a ladder fall, and has received paid sick leave while you have been out for childbirth and received no compensation, you probably have grounds for a pregnancy-based claim.

If someone asks when you are leaving—or whether or not you have plans to leave—and indicates that he or she wants your job, this is *not* discrimination. This is being a creep, but it is not discrimination.

Being denied a promotion because of pregnancy is very difficult to prove unless you automatically receive a promotion on the annual anniversary of your hiring date and you are denied one while pregnant.

Fear of Filing a Complaint

Many women are aware that they are not treated equitably, yet are reluctant to talk about their feelings with their employers or to file a discrimination charge. Eleanor Holmes Norton, former head of the Equal Employment Opportunity Commission, the federal agency that enforces civil-rights law, says to "assume you have rights. This [pregnancy-based discrimination] is a developing field," Norton says. "It is not yet in place, and women are entitled to know what their rights are."

There are several reasons why women are reluctant to file charges:

- They lack knowledge about their rights and the laws already available to them.

- It's unpleasant.

- It may be years before the case comes to trial.

- The woman might lose the case.

- It may be expensive.

- They fear retaliation by the employer.

Many women also feel "grateful" that they are allowed to work during their pregnancies, and not that it is their right to do so.

Other women feel guilty when they take time off to have a child, rationalizing that this is a burden to place on an employer. Others feel guilty when they return to their jobs, because of the traditional view that a mother's place is in the home.

Fear of retaliation, however, is most often the reason women are reluctant to fight for equal treatment on the job. For many women there is always the concern that if you rock the boat, somewhere that charge is going to catch up with you. You may never know how a potential employer or colleague hears about you. It may be over dinner at the country club. It may be during a tennis game. Or it may come from someone's wife who is having lunch with someone who knows you. Most working women know that the work network is pretty small but the ripples are pretty large. And like it or not, a discrimination charge may not only affect your current job but haunt your career path in the years ahead.

Try to Settle Your Complaint In-House

Before you file a discrimination charge with a state or federal agency, try to settle your complaint through whatever in-house procedures exist.

Many employers simply do not know how to handle a working pregnancy and may not have faced the situation enough times to have developed a standard policy regarding pregnant employees. You might approach your employer by indicating that you are bringing this situation to his attention in an effort to make things better for the future, that it's a situation he will probably have to face sooner or later, and that you have a genuine desire to remain at your job and help develop an equitable solution for *all* parties concerned. Before you do any talking, however, do the following:

- *Write down what you think your case is before you discuss it with anyone.* Review the events, the people involved, any conversations that took place, and determine exactly what it is that you want resolved. Is it on-the-job treatment? Elimination of mandatory leave policies (illegal since a Supreme Court decision in 1974)? Temporary disability benefits during your absence from the job? Gather any written materials available in case you require documentation of your situation.

- *Assess the situation as objectively as possible.* You may have to go through a bit of soul-searching to determine whether this is something you really want to do, because of its effects over the long term. You may decide to take action, but you might also consider that a male employee with a physical disability would probably not file a complaint under similar circumstances.

  Because of the nature of the working world, you may win the victory but lose the war. You may be accused of not being a team player and of not being company oriented. In fact, your boss may view you with suspicion for even bringing up the subject.

- *Ask yourself a variety of objective questions.* These include,

Where are you in your career? What is your standing in the company? Are you good enough to get a job with another company? How is the job market? What are your plans after the baby is born? How long have you been with the company? Have they been sensitive to this type of complaint before? How many women at the office have been pregnant before you, and what has their experience at the company been? What type of company is it? Conservative? Progressive?

- *Talk to someone you trust, and who can keep quiet until you have made a decision, to make certain that your views are objective.* Among the questions you should discuss are, Do you have anyone to defend or support you? What do you think the reaction will be if you should decide to file a complaint?

  Analyze what the possibilities of retaliation are. You might lose your job—either now or in the future. What does this mean to you in terms of dollars and cents? Aside from salary, what types of benefits have you accumulated during your time with the company?

  After you have done this, you are then ready to approach your employer.

- *Make a complaint to the appropriate in-house person or to your superior.* State your case clearly—and verbally. Do not provide anything in writing at this point. You can talk from your own notes. State your facts and explain what has happened in detail. You might say that you do not believe this is right, that it may be against the law, and you wanted to talk about it with your employer first.

  One teacher who was initially denied tenure due to a six-week break for maternity leave fought the decision and won. She later heard the superintendent of schools say to her principal, "Frankly, we were concerned that she was going to go to the Civil Liberties Union." The teacher admitted that this would have been her next step if the complaint had not been resolved in her favor.

  After you have stated your case, wait to see how your employer responds to you.

- *Expect some defensive action from your employer.* He may ignore you, or he may harass or ridicule you in hopes that you will leave. He might move you out of your office, pass the word not to give you any work because you don't plan to return after the birth of the baby, overload you with work, or indicate that you are not performing up to par.

He may tell you that your perception of the situation is unclear in hopes that you assume the defensive position rather than the offensive one. He may also insinuate that your strained emotional state has caused you to get your facts confused.

He may also use the argument that your pregnancy is a "voluntary" situation and is therefore not to be considered in the same classification as other temporary disabilities. DON'T BELIEVE IT! Confront this argument with the fact that it is a discrimination problem, not a voluntary condition. If your employer provides for certain policies and benefits for other temporary physical disabilities, he is lawfully obligated to provide equal treatment for his pregnant employees.

Stand by your belief that you are being discriminated against if you have reason to believe you are! Trust your instincts. But don't prematurely anticipate a negative reaction from your employer, and don't discount the possibility that he may agree with you and move to change the company's policy.

If you have no success in filing a complaint in-house, then consider another approach. If your talks end in no action after a reasonable amount of time, you may consider seeing a lawyer—either through legal aid or by hiring a private one. Have your lawyer write a *tactful* letter to your employer, stating the situation and indicating that it *may* be in violation of the law. You might have your lawyer add that before invoking any state or federal statutes you would like to have the opportunity to talk about the situation. If your employer is at all sensitive to outside interference, he will probably want to listen to your complaints at this point. If you still receive no satisfaction, then you may want to consider pursuing your complaint through a state or federal agency.

If you are one person with an individual problem, negotiating a complaint may be easier, because there may be fewer hard feelings involved. Your employer may also be more willing to make an exception to the rule rather than change his company policies for the future.

However, if you are dealing with a situation involving many women and your employer is reluctant to change his policies, you may feel it is important enough to garner support among other female employees in the same situation and consider filing a class action suit. (But do not conduct strategy sessions on company time!) Your employer may be less likely to retaliate if there is more than one person filing the complaint, and he or she may be less apt to try to discredit the group as a whole. You will also have more resources available and more support in a group, especially in a union. Furthermore, class action suits tend to make court access easier.

● *Whatever you decide, stay enthusiastic and continue to perform your job responsibilities to the best of your capabilities.* If you are unsuccessful in settling your complaint within your company structure, you can go to an outside agency. There are several ways of doing this—particularly through the union grievance procedure or through a state or federal human-rights agency. Specific guidelines for filing a charge through either of these methods are detailed in the appendix on pages 245–53.

Occupational Safety: A Knotty Question

Occupational safety becomes a discrimination issue when employers refuse to hire women of childbearing age on the grounds that exposure to toxic substances may be harmful to their reproductive systems, or when pregnant women are transferred to positions that are usually safer but also lower paying. In some instances, women who request transfers to safer jobs during pregnancy may be denied their request, thus forcing the woman to choose between her and her baby's health and her paycheck. Occupational safety for the pregnant woman is a double-edged sword.

At this point there are no answers. There is a lack of information, a lack of administrative guidelines and no consistent court decisions about the issue. Furthermore, industry does not fully attack the problems of occupational health because of the eventual costs of cleaning up the work environment. It is certain, however, that there will be changes in the future.

Former Equal Employment Opportunity Commissioner Eleanor Holmes Norton describes the question of occupational hazards as "one of the great frontier issues under Title VII." The issues involving occupational safety and the pregnant woman are complex, but what they come down to is whether the exclusion of pregnant women from any job is discriminatory.

The Equal Employment Opportunity Commission is currently working with two other federal agencies, the Occupational Safety and Health Administration (OSHA) and the National Institute for Occupational Safety and Health (NIOSH), in studying this problem. They are beginning to make recommendations about what may be considered discriminatory. If you have any concerns or questions, check with the OSHA or NIOSH offices listed in the appendix on pages 227–30, or with your union.

Because this is a developing issue, employers are responding in a variety of ways. Most are aware that certain substances are risky. The employer will usually inform employees of the risk and safety precautions involved. It is up to the individual to make the decision whether to accept or reject the job.

Because most of the women affected by occupational hazards are employed in industrial positions, the unions play a unique role in this issue. The United Auto Workers' policy, for instance, is that the union has a joint responsibility with the employer to explain potential hazards to an employee, but it is up to the employee to make the decision whether or not to work. Odessa Komer, director of the UAW Woman's Department, said that an informal "informed consent" by female UAW workers to work under an occupationally hazardous situation was necessary.

Although many unions feel that this issue should be dealt with through Congress and OSHA, others feel that it should be a collective-bargaining issue. But the trade union position, in general, has been that health hazards are equally unsafe for women and men, and the answer is to clean up the work place rather than discriminate. Sylvia Krekel, an occupational health specialist at the Oil, Chemical and Atomic Workers Union, said that the trend for the future would be to demand remedies through both the collective-bargaining process and the law.

Krekel said that a woman who finds herself in a situation where she is exposed to toxic substances should ask to be transferred to a less hazardous position on a temporary basis, but with full economic protection, including maintenance of seniority and pay. This should be done with union backing. Because this is a new issue, however, you may not get very far if you request such conditions. You will, however, be bringing the issue to light.

Talk with other women—and men—who are considering having children. Approach your union representative as a group, and try to go through the union grievance procedure explained in the appendix on pages 249–53. You might also contact your local EEOC office as well as your regional OSHA or NIOSH office. (See the appendix for the listing.) You should be aware, however, that this is one area where industry has been more successful than employees.

The End of Pregnancy-Based Discrimination

Pregnancy-based discrimination is just the beginning of what must be changed in the revolution of attitudes toward working women and reproduction. Women are not going to stop having babies, nor are they likely to become less active in the labor force.

The area of rights for the pregnant woman is in flux. By questioning common employment practices that limit opportunities or benefits due to pregnancy, you can help others recognize that pregnancy should not be a barrier to women in the work place nor an economic burden for their families. There are four basic ways to protect your rights during pregnancy: voluntary compliance by your employer, the political process, collective bargaining agreements, and court decisions. All are dependent upon action by you. Question whatever inequities you feel exist, and work to eliminate them. The tools are accessible— use them.

THE MEANING OF YOUR WORKING PREGNANCY

Your pregnancy means more than nine months of gestation on the job. It means that the pregnant woman who works has a support group available to her today that wasn't there a few years ago—and this constituency can help to change attitudes, not only for the pregnant woman who is trying to be an active part of the work force, but for all women who are confronted with the mother-versus-worker role. The working pregnant woman can visibly demonstrate that it is possible for a woman to consider combining two very important aspects of her life—a career and children.

In an era when a pregnant newscaster can broadcast the news throughout her pregnancy, when pregnant lawyers can appear in court, when a teacher can use her expanding belly as a lesson in human growth and development, we can no longer assume that pregnancy means the end of a career and a retreat from the world.

2

TAKING CHARGE OF YOUR MEDICAL CARE

Every pregnant woman has a right to the very best that the medical system has to offer. Whether or not you receive quality care—from the start of your pregnancy through delivery to your postpartum checkup—depends on a certain savvy, information, and your own readiness to make the medical system work for you and your baby.

In seeking and demanding quality care you have more power than you may think, because you are the consumer in a nation where health service is the third largest industry and where obstetrics is a very competitive business. With a decline in the birth rate and a rise in the number of competitors—midwives and family practitioners (a modern version of the old-fashioned family doctor)—obstetricians and maternity hospitals have to be responsive to consumer wishes.

Your own power as a consumer seeking the kind of maternity services you want is magnified because of a revolution in the American way of birth. This change, demanded by women, childbirth activists and concerned medical professionals, has led to a well-publicized emphasis on family-centered obstetrics. No longer is the physician in solitary and unquestioned command except in matters of safety. At a major clinical meeting, for example, the American College of Obstetricians and Gynecologists scheduled a debate entitled, "Who's Running the Show?" There was discussion but no debate, because it

38

was clear that the woman is the key person in her own pregnancy.

Active participation in your own medical care during pregnancy may be the last thing that you—and perhaps your doctor—want. But it is absolutely essential. You and your baby are too important to be entrusted totally to others. Furthermore, we found in our interviews with pregnant women, concerned physicians, and childbirth activists and in important studies that the medical aspects of pregnancy, childbirth and hospital care in the United States vary greatly.

There are at least three important reasons why you should participate in your medical care. First, active involvement will help keep you in control during these nine special months of your life. Up until now, women have handed total control over to the medical profession and this has caused such resentment and anger that it is no surprise that obstetrics and gynecology have been prime targets of the women's movement for self-advancement and respect.

Second, you need to select, monitor and question your care, because in obstetrics there are no guarantees; no physician is perfect. You owe it to yourself, and to your baby, to demand the best. Medical science has the capability of identifying approximately two thirds of the high risk babies *before* birth through prenatal screening, evaluation and testing. Equally important, with the right care even an infant weighing less than two and a half pounds has a 40 percent chance of *healthy* survival. You may not need it, but you will want access to that kind of medical expertise.

Third, you have to decide just what you want and you must work to get it, because there is a collision between advanced modern technology and the age-old process of normal childbirth. We will spotlight controversies about such matters as fetal heart monitoring, elective induction of labor and the use of diagnostic ultrasound, which are generally referred to as "technological intervention" in the natural process of childbirth. We will present alternative options in prenatal and childbirth care. If you haven't yet decided what medical care is right for you, we can give you facts to help shape your decision. If you are already receiving care, we can help you assess its quality. We will also sketch a very current and important revision of the entire maternity hospital picture in the United States.

There are many fine books readily available that detail your childbirth options. We don't want to duplicate these books and we don't want to dictate. There is no right or wrong way to have your baby. There are, however, variations in the quality of prenatal and childbirth care. It is our goal to help you receive the best. We hope to enable you to participate in your care with knowledge and without strain. Your pregnancy months are not a battlefield, but you do have to work out what you want from your maternity care team and what you can reasonably expect. Labor is no time to discover that you and your doctor have differing views on childbirth.

As a patient, as a woman, as a pregnant woman, you may have trouble dealing with the medical world. There are reasons why. We will look at these reasons through the experiences of pregnant women we have interviewed. Then we will suggest ways to modify your thinking and behavior to give clear signals that you expect to be treated well.

If you need a chuckle—or some rage—to make you glad that the world has changed enough so that you *are* part of your care, scan these excerpts from 1952, when *McCall's* magazine asked twelve obstetricians, who together delivered a total of 2,500 babies a year, to express their views for an article entitled "What Your Obstetrician Thinks of You." The following three pregnant patient "types" were on the doctors' all-time "lemon" list:

"*The Shopper*—who markets for an obstetrician the way she does for a choice head of lettuce. Going from one doctor to another, she compares notes on personal appearance, office decor, hospital connections, preference in anesthesia, fees and clientele . . . we like to assume the patient has decided, 'this is my doctor,' and is ready to let him take over.

"*The Know-It-All*—picks up her knowledge over the clothesline, at bridge parties and at her mother's knee." She has the audacity to quiz her doctor "on vitamins, drugs, measurements, breech births, Caesareans, forceps, rooming-in and Rh, [and] she proceeds to instruct him in *her* methods.

"*The Cipher*" is either too silent or too passive to express herself. "You feel as if you might as well be practicing plumbing as medicine," one obstetrician said in an interview.

The magazine noted that "in every instance, the patient the doctor likes best and finds easiest to work with is the one who likes and trusts him . . . one doctor said that he finds the 'good' patient is usually healthy, intelligent, well balanced, happily married, not too curious about her body, with little time or inclination to worry about herself and a strong desire to have a baby." One doctor who happened to like race horses said, "I like that kind of woman—smart looking, high strung, quick on the trigger." Another favored women who had trouble conceiving, because they were so grateful.

If you have any personal doubt that women—yourself included—have influenced the medical world, think whether any obstetrician, let alone twelve prominent ones, would allow those quotes in print today! It is important to like and trust your doctor, but the day of the passive, docile, unquestioning "good" patient is over. We are all on the "lemon" list, and it is a fine place to be.

The challenge of making the medical system work for you and your baby is a sizable one. The more facts at your command, the easier your task will be.

Just What Is "Quality Care"?

The vast majority of pregnancies are normal, with successful results. That is something your health care team will probably tell you as soon as you ask. If there are problems, they usually occur in these ways: (1) A woman starts pregnancy with a medical problem, such as heart disease; (2) she develops a pregnancy complication, such as hypertension; or (3) after a normal pregnancy a complication occurs during labor or delivery. Although it is not likely that you'll have a problem, it is because of these possibilities that you need continuous high-quality care as soon as you suspect that you are pregnant. Particularly in the early weeks of pregnancy, you need a professional with whom to discuss any drugs that you are taking and to raise the question of genetic testing or of any modifications in your work or daily habits.

High-quality obstetrical care means careful and continuous surveillance—from the early pregnancy months through delivery to postpartum checkup—by trained professionals who know that pregnancy and delivery are normal physiological events, but who are also alert to potential problems, are able to recognize them as early as possible, and can deal with them or call in an expert. High-quality obstetrical care means access to the best facilities possible, and in some instances it means making sure that a woman is in such a facility before a high-risk baby is born.

High-quality obstetrical care means something else— it means treating the pregnant woman as an individual worthy of respect and personal attention. It means planning a woman's care with her, using understandable terms—and doing this not as a benevolent favor, but in the name of good care.

AN ADDED DIMENSION OF QUALITY CARE

Every age and every culture has its own definition of what constitutes quality obstetrical care. Queen Victoria, for example, was delighted to learn about chloroform to ease childbirth pains. For decades thereafter women looked to medication for help, and accepted it gratefully. Many of us were born in the haze of our mothers' "twilight sleep," while our fathers were banished to waiting rooms to pace for hours, becoming the unhappy subjects of cartoons and jokes.

Today, husbands are allowed in the delivery room in many hospitals. It may be possible for you to be thoroughly awake and active in childbirth; and rather than be whisked away to an impersonal nursery, your new baby may be cuddled minutes after birth and kept close to you throughout your hospital stay. This tremendous changeover is still far from complete, which means that you may have to fight for the kind of childbirth you want.

The fight began in the early 1930's, when Dr. Grantly

Dick Read initiated his publications on natural childbirth. The most famous, *Childbirth Without Fear,* was published in 1944. By 1950, the first natural childbirth association in the United States was formed in Milwaukee. Soon other groups formed. Then in 1959 an American named Marjorie Karmel published *Thank You, Dr. Lamaze,* describing her childbirth experience using the method of a French physician, Dr. Fernand Lamaze. A year later the International Childbirth Education Association was formed in the United States. By 1978 it had some 12,000 members. In addition to the ICEA, there are other parents' groups, some of which call for an even more radical alternative to traditional hospital delivery— home delivery.

Meanwhile, establishment obstetrics has endorsed the concept of family-centered obstetrics. Since this concept covers matters that may be appealing or important to you, it is worth a close-up look.

FAMILY-CENTERED OBSTETRICS

Family-centered obstetrics works from a different starting point than traditional obstetrics. In essence, its argument is that instead of the pregnant woman being considered in isolation, the expectant family—father, the other children, even the grandparents—should be involved in the pregnancy in a meaningful way. Family-centered obstetricians say that a family begins to form or regroup itself for a new member before birth. By approaching the total pregnancy experience together, the outcome will be better for mother, father and offspring. In seeking quality care or in assessing what you are already receiving, you can see whether attention to this concept is or should be part of your care.

Family-centered obstetrics is so highly rated that a wide variety of professional groups and parents' organizations has recommended that each hospital in the country set up representative committees to balance the demand for family-centered care with the hospital's staff, capabilities and facilities.

Family-centered obstetrics means a willingness on the

part of your physician to include your husband and, perhaps, your other children in at least one prenatal visit; it means encouragement for the childbearing couple to attend prepared childbirth classes, and a true desire to help them deliver their child with as little medication or intervention as is safely possible.

"Since it takes a couple to create a new life in the first place, the father's participation in labor and delivery, rather than being denied, should be actively sought. Every day seems to bring forth new evidence of the potential value of this initial bonding of the mother, father, and child," says Dr. Richard H. Aubry, professor of obstetrics and gynecology, State University of New York at Syracuse, and chairman of District II of the American College of Obstetricians and Gynecologists.

Comments Mrs. Doris Olson of Minneapolis, a past president of the International Childbirth Education Association, "My initial childbirth occurred while I was drugged, half there, half not there, somewhat out of my mind. I just sort of observed the whole thing. Of course, my husband wasn't there. I don't say that we love our oldest child any the less, but the way that our other children were born without drugs, with my husband there to help, made an immediate difference."

Family-centered obstetrics symbolizes a theme important to you, however and wherever you deliver, all through the pregnancy months: Childbearing is your experience; it is not the property of the medical profession.

Your search for the best in obstetrical care means finding professionals with sound training and human sensitivity, and you might keep the idea of family-centered obstetrics as an additional criterion. It is far easier to define the quality of proper obstetrical care than to find it—not because it doesn't exist, but because there are so many options, variations and choices.

YOUR OPTIONS IN OBSTETRICAL CARE

For most women, obstetrical care means a doctor/patient relationship. Although anyone with an M.D. degree is legally allowed to deliver babies, not everyone should.

Some hospitals won't permit doctors without special qualification to admit obstetrical patients.

The most qualified specialist is a board-certified Fellow of the American College of Obstetricians and Gynecologists who has had a high level of postgraduate training and experience and who has passed a rigorous examination. The ACOG encourages its 22,000 members to develop their expertise and capabilities through continuing medical education. This is a plus for patients.

Other obstetricians in your community may be *board eligible,* which means that they meet requirements of the College but have not yet passed the necessary examination. Still other physicians call themselves gynecologists or obstetricians and women's health may be their entire practice, but they may have had only courses in these fields. Osteopathic physicians also do obstetrical care.

There is also a growing trend in the United States towards the establishment of family practice as a medical specialty. Essentially, the family practitioner is a revival of the old-fashioned family doctor, one who takes care of all health problems the same way that the pediatrician takes total care of the child's health. A board-certified family practitioner may have taken a brief special curriculum in obstetrics designed by ACOG.

For many women, obstetrical care involves a group medical practice, which means seeing various members of the group on prenatal visits, any one of whom can deliver the child. Some women view this as a plus that eliminates the old problem, "What if my doctor is on vacation when I go into labor?" There is a growing trend toward prepaid total medical care through the so-called HMO, health maintenance organization. If you are in such a plan and want to use it for maternity care, it is a cost advantage. However, you will have to use an obstetrician who has been prechosen, and not by you.

As for well-trained female obstetricians, while many pregnant women would like to use them, there were only about two thousand female members of ACOG in the United States in 1980, although, according to Dr. Warren Pearse, executive director of ACOG, this situation is rapidly changing. In a 1978 interview he said, "At present, twenty-five percent of our residents are women and if this trend continues—and we expect it to—one fifth of all obstetrician-gynecologists will be women in twelve years." Some female obstetrician-gynecologists have advanced attitudes; others have fought so long and hard to be accepted by the male obstetrical establishment that they may mirror traditional male attitudes. But if nothing else, female obstetrician-gynecologists know what it is like to be a working woman.

THE TEAM APPROACH IN OBSTETRICS

Although the doctor/patient relationship is the one the public automatically associates with maternal care, such care is actually a team approach. For example, there are thousands of registered nurses in this country with special training, experience and, recently, certification by the Nurses' Association of ACOG, which qualifies them as very skilled professionals in obstetrical-gynecological nursing. Although they work as adjuncts to physicians, they have many important responsibilities, including preliminary screening of pregnant women in prenatal clinics and care and monitoring of almost all pregnant women in labor and delivery.

These nurses are involved in research to improve maternal and newborn health. They educate women, and perhaps most important, they bring a special interest and attention to the emotional and social aspects of childbearing. They are, therefore, important to all of us. In addition, trained ob-gyn nurses can help you learn how to care for your body after childbirth and for your demanding newborn.

Other professionals you should know about—but may not think of—are hospital social workers, who may help you ease family problems and arrange such help as, for example, a visiting nurse service for when you come home. Much more obvious sources of information and help are the childbirth educators prominent in many communities. They may be nurses or specially trained people able to teach exercises that will help you prepare your body for labor. They may also conduct classes where you and your husband can learn how to deliver your baby in as relaxed and drug-free a manner as possible.

Some parent preparation classes are held in homes, some in hospitals, some in physicians' offices. These classes are useful because they put you in contact with other couples living the pregnancy experience, a contact that can continue long after delivery and can be a great help in coping with life with a newborn. However you deliver, these classes are designed to ease the mystery and fear of the childbirth experience. In some areas your other children may be invited to attend these classes. This offers yet another way to make childbearing a true family event.

These prenatal classes are worth the extra cost for many reasons. They can (1) teach you the early signs of labor and what to do; (2) preview what will happen in the hospital and take you on a tour of the facilities, so that when you arrive you will be in familiar surroundings; (3) offer you a chance to share the pregnancy experience with your husband; (4) enable you to meet other couples in your community and to set up valuable contacts for mutual support and information; and (5) educate you about childbirth medications.

Not all childbirth classes are great. Not all instructors are perfect. Many, however, are interested and enthusiastic people who can add an element of friendship to an impersonal hospital setting. If a childbirth education class is not all that you hoped, you may have to shop around and find another.

In choosing a childbirth education program keep in mind the fact there are different methods of prepared childbirth. For questions about different approaches check with an ICEA chapter in your area or the main office listed in the appendix.

Prepared childbirth classes have a small drawback. They tend to lead you to expect a drug-free ecstatic childbirth experience, which you may have; but in obstetrics, as we said, there are no guarantees. You may need procedures that you would rather avoid. It is truly important for you to remember that the experience of childbirth is not the supreme test of you as a person. If it turns out that for one reason or another your experience is a disappointment, don't feel guilty. That kind of reaction can only hurt you. To avoid it, don't expect too much. Also, never try to compete with anyone else's obstetrical performance.

A NEW OLD OPTION: MIDWIFERY

A new option in the spectrum of health care today comes from a very welcome emerging group—certified nurse-midwives. Although midwifery accounts for the delivery of only one percent of all births in the United States in the late 1970's, training is on the increase and there is a growing demand for midwives. The American College of Nurse-Midwives has been established, headquartered in Washington, D.C., and certified nurse-midwives who have met rigorous requirements are officially recognized by the American College of Obstetricians and Gynecologists. These are professionals trained in the skills of midwifery; they are not "grannies" or "lay midwives," women who have decided to designate themselves as birth attendants.

A nurse-midwife is trained to provide complete prenatal care and to help women deliver their babies in the most natural way possible. They can monitor and be responsible for normal pregnancies only, but can recognize potential problems and arrange expert assistance. Since most nurse-midwives are women, they bring their experience and knowledge as women to professional obstetrical care. Many nurse-midwives may have started their careers as obstetrical nurses, and in some parts of the country they are totally responsible for prenatal care and delivery; if everything goes well, a pregnant woman may never see an M.D.

Early in this century midwife deliveries were common in this country—as they are today abroad. However, with the growth of a rich, powerful male obstetrical establishment, American midwives were virtually driven out of existence. Whether fairly or not, midwives were characterized as ignorant and superstitious, and as agents of infection that killed many mothers and children. Professional midwives were allowed a comeback to help care for poor women in pregnancy and labor; ironically, it is the private obstetrical patient who is now enthusiastically seeking nurse-midwife care. Midwifery may again flourish in this country.

An example of this new trend can be found at Roosevelt Hospital in New York City. In 1977, 253 pregnant women, mostly white, almost all married, the majority with college-plus graduate degrees, found their way to Roosevelt. These pregnant women—nurses, lawyers, doctors, sociologists, secretaries, students—all of whom could command top-level traditional obstetrical care, were seeking something else: pregnancy and childbirth support, comfort, guidance from another woman and no interference in the normal body process.

"The midwives' role is not authoritarian, but one of friend-adviser," explained Barbara Brennan, C.N.M. (certified nurse-midwife), leader of the Roosevelt program and coauthor of *The Complete Book of Midwifery*. "We make a point of sharing everything with our clients. We never do anything to them; rather, we do things with them, explaining our position and our thoughts every step of the way. We are willing to consider any ideas or demands they may have concerning their own childbirth, and we bend to them whenever possible."

In 1964 Ms. Brennan was one of the first women in the United States educated and certified a nurse-midwife. When she went to work at Roosevelt, she was assigned to clinic patients. Slowly, professional respect for what she was doing grew, and in 1974, with four other certified nurse-midwives and the encouragement of Dr. Thomas Dillon, director, Obstetrics and Gynecology Services at Roosevelt Hospital in New York City, Ms. Brennan opened a group practice within the hospital.

Midwives don't call pregnant women "patients." The word "patient" is derived from the verb *patior,* which means "to suffer." Midwives don't see pregnancy as an illness or a cause of suffering. Midwives call pregnant women "clients," and some pregnant women know and appreciate what they are buying. After explaining that they will handle only normal, low-risk pregnancies, certified nurse-midwives make this promise: You will never be left alone in labor.

"Our clients also know that they can call us with any question," Barbara Brennan said. "They call us more

freely than they would a physician. If they don't feel the
baby move for a few hours, or they are worried about the
effect on the baby of painting the ceiling, they call. We
encourage them to bring in questions."

At first, insurance companies did not want to cover
midwifery services. Now many do. "Blue Shield here in
New York didn't want to have anything to do with us,"
Ms. Brennan said, "but recently there was a newspaper
story that the Federal Trade Commission was going after
companies that created a monopoly by paying only doctors' fees. Blue Shield couldn't get a meeting with us
started fast enough!"

The word about midwifery is getting out. In some
areas—for example, Americus, Georgia—obstetricians are
in joint practice with nurse-midwives. An obstetrician
who moved into a new town soon discovered that he was
at a competitive disadvantage while practicing solo. When
a thirty-year-old nurse-midwife went to work in an obstetrical group practice in upstate New York, every doctor and nurse in town watched her with suspicion, while
women asked, "Why didn't I have this kind of care for
my first delivery?"

THE SUPERPROFESSIONALS
AND GENETIC SERVICES

The superspecialists are perinatologists, who specialize in
managing hish-risk pregnancies, and neonatologists, pediatricians who work with high-risk newborns. These highly
trained people are few in number and are usually located
at large teaching hospitals.

If you have medical complications, develop a complication of pregnancy or have had obstetrical problems in the
past, you may want to be under the care of a perinatologist,
who has access to advanced diagnostic techniques and
equipment. A perinatologist will monitor you during pregnancy and will be in charge of labor and delivery.
Perinatologists also act as consultants to less-specialized
obstetricians in the community.

As we noted earlier, many problems in newborns can at
least be apprehended during pregnancy. It is part of

quality care that your obstetrician make sure that a pediatrician or neonatologist will be available when your child is born. Usually the decision to call in experts is made by your obstetrician. However, if you have had other children with problems, even such a slight one as slow development, you should question your family pediatrician. Sometimes problems can be traced back to an occurrence during pregnancy or childbirth that can be avoided in another pregnancy.

If, after birth, your newborn seems to be having any problem, you should demand immediate expert attention. Don't "wait and see." Sometimes this may mean that you must be in one hospital while your baby goes to another, but even this separation is tolerable if intensive care is needed. Usually the staff of intensive-care nurseries is highly sensitive to the feelings of parents and should help you maintain contact with your baby.

Fortunately, most women don't need the care of superspecialists. But two general groups of candidates for extra care include pregnant teen-agers and women over thirty-five. Through federal and state bureaus, health agencies (such as the March of Dimes Birth Defects Foundation), and community service groups, there are programs to help the pregnant teen-ager. If you are over thirty-five, however, there is less clear information about just what you require.

Many women interviewed for this book were in their thirties; a few were older. Age is not a barrier to a healthy pregnancy and successful outcome. You do, however, want expert obstetrical care, from either a board-certified obstetrician or a perinatologist, because older women have a higher risk of medical complications, such as diabetes or kidney disease. Older women also may have problems in labor and delivery that require special attention. An older woman, for example, may be more likely to need a cesarean section.

Amniocentesis

Amniocentesis is a procedure in which a small amount of fluid is removed from the womb. This fluid sample is then subjected to a variety of laboratory tests, one of which can spot Down's syndrome (mongolism). The incidence of this severe birth defect increases in proportion to a pregnant woman's age. This is the greatest birth-defect risk of an older pregnancy, and fortunately it can be detected.

Amniocentesis has been performed on many thousands of pregnant women in this country and abroad. It is undoubtedly a valuable diagnostic tool. Because older pregnant women—those over thirty-five—do have a greater Down's syndrome risk, and because a physician who fails to recommend proper genetic testing may be liable for heavy financial damages if a detectable but neglected birth defect occurs, amniocentesis is often a routine matter for women over thirty-five.

However, studies in Great Britain and elsewhere suggest that because of risks, though very slight, to the baby and mother, it may be advisable to suggest amniocentesis only for pregnant women at age forty and above, unless a young woman has a suspicious family history or has borne or miscarried a child with a defect.

Amniocentesis is something to discuss with your medical team so that you can insist on a full explanation of any possible risk. If you decide to have the procedure, it is wise to select an expert, the person who has had a great deal of experience in doing the technique.

Please note that this discussion centers on midpregnancy amniocentesis for genetic diagnostic purposes. As you approach childbirth, amniocentesis may be done to determine the health of your baby. That is a different matter altogether.

Regardless of your age, if you know—or even just think—that there has been an inherited disease or defect in your family or your husband's, you should discuss this matter with your physician as soon as possible. Among detectable genetic diseases are sickle-cell anemia (most common among black people), Tay-Sachs disease (most common among Jews of Eastern European ancestry) and phenylketonuria, a metabolic disorder.

Medical genetic services are usually located at medical centers or teaching hospitals. Often these services work on a physician-referral basis only. These services can do laboratory tests, offer diagnoses and give counsel about pregnancy and newborn treatment. For information about available services, check with your local March of Dimes chapter. You should also know that the Foundation has professional information available to your doctor, and that there are "outreach" programs, which give your physician access to experts. This means that even if you live in an isolated community you can get assistance for genetic problems.

WHERE BABIES ARE BORN—
THE HOSPITAL SCENE

We have described the various medical professionals important to your pregnancy. Before we can offer suggestions about how to determine the kind of care that is right and comfortable for you, we have to look at hospitals. The overwhelming majority of American babies are born in the hospital; a few are born in specialized maternity centers; and there are no true statistics on the others—the number of babies born at home or where their mothers happen to be. These facts may change, but not yet.

As a pregnant woman, you don't choose just a physician; you also choose the hospital with which he or she is affiliated, an institution with rules and attitudes of its own. This means that you have to learn what services the hospitals in your community offer and what their philosophy of childbirth may be. We will suggest some questions to help you size up your hospitals.

First, however, you should know that a major reorganization of maternity care is underway in U.S. hospitals. This reorganization is considered necessary, not only to improve the U.S. maternity health record but also to put a lid on skyrocketing medical costs by making the best use of professionals and medical resources, such as neonatal intensive-care units. This plan has the endorsement of the March of Dimes Birth Defects Foundation, the American Academy of Family Physicians, the American Academy of Pediatrics, the American Medical Association and the American College of Obstetricians and Gynecologists. It is criticized by those in rural areas who have staged protests to keep local hospitals from being shut, and by

health activists who claim it reduces the options in deciding where to have a baby and makes intervention more
likely.

Essentially, the reorganization creates three different
types of maternity facilities:

● A "level-I hospital" is the simplest facility, equipped to provide prenatal care for low-risk maternity cases and normal
  deliveries. Professional nurses have large responsibilities, and
  certified nurse-midwives can take care of normal deliveries
  under the supervision of a physician.

● A "level-II hospital" is bigger and has more specialized personnel and equipment. For example, this hospital can usually
  do a cesarean section on an emergency basis within fifteen
  minutes; it should have a special nursery for mildly ill infants,
  and a special unit for severely ill newborns where they can be
  treated prior to transport to the next kind of hospital.

● A "level-III hospital" is a superhospital, handling thousands
  of normal and high-risk births each year and serving as the
  most specialized facility within a region. The experts at this
  facility are supposed to educate, consult with and help professionals in surrounding communities.

The three-level hospital organization works on the theory that it is the responsibility of the local physician,
nurse-midwife, obstetrician-gynecologist—and level-I
hospitals—to evaluate all pregnant women for high-risk
potential, and to make referrals or ask for consultation
when necessary. According to Dr. Arthur J. Salisbury,
vice-president of medical services of the March of Dimes,
the three-level plan either is being effected or is in late
planning stages in every state.

As a pregnant woman you must learn what is available
in your area, and if there should be problems, where the
nearest level-III hospital is. A level-I hospital may be just
right for a normal delivery close to home; the same with a
level-II. But for problems, level-III is where you want to
be. In your community "regional" maternity care organization may be the term used instead of "level" but the
idea is the same. Just inform yourself about the special
capabilities of hospitals in your area and neighboring
ones.

HOW TO ASSESS A HOSPITAL

For your own benefit and that of your family and your new baby, it is useful to evaluate a hospital (whatever its level) in terms of its provisions for family-centered care. Some hospitals are traditional and ignore these matters. Others offer at least some of the aspects of a warm, supportive atmosphere. There can be great differences between hospitals in the same community. Here are some questions to ask:

Does the hospital have, offer or permit

- Prepared childbirth classes that emphasize the avoidance of excessive medication?

- Hospital tours, including the labor-and-delivery rooms; maternal exercise classes; instruction in the care of the newborn for both parents?

- Fathers to participate throughout labor and delivery as long as it is safely possible? In the event of a cesarean, can the pregnant woman be kept awake and the father be present if they both wish?

- A physical environment conducive to a family event—that is, is there a "birthing room," a multipurpose labor and recovery room with homelike decor (rocking chairs and so forth) where normal deliveries can take place?

- Do both the mother and father have a chance to hold their newborn right after delivery? Is the family quickly separated after birth? Is the infant accessible to both parents on a twenty-four-hour basis? Are the couple's other children allowed to visit their mother and new brother or sister?

- Is there help and support for women who wish to breast-feed?

- Is the hospital stay as short as possible—twenty-four to thirty-six hours if both mother and child are doing well?

- If a baby needs intensive care, can parents visit and help feed or bathe their child? What happens if an infant is transferred to a special facility in another hospital?

Whether you are forced to use a particular hospital because of your doctor's affiliation or your medical needs, or you are assessing hospitals in your area before making a choice of doctor, it is always vital to ask about the nursing staff and ratio of labor-and-delivery nurses to the usual patient load. You can ask this question of your physician, the labor-and-delivery nursing supervisor or a hospital administrator before you have need of the hospital services. The nurse-patient ratio is important to determine, because many pregnant women worry that they will be left alone during labor. The ideal ratio is one nurse for every woman in labor. If this is not possible, ask what the usual ratio is and what happens when the labor-and-delivery floor becomes very busy. Hospital personnel have a very good idea of staff ratio to work flow. If you think that the hospital you have in mind tends to be understaffed, you might consider another.

Hospitals depend on the public for business. Consumer pressure—the use of a particular hospital because it offers good service—is a powerful persuader. In some communities, mothers' groups have convinced hospitals to develop the kind of maternity facilities they want. Childbirth educators and women who have recently given birth are excellent sources for a realistic appraisal of hospitals in your community. In addition, in some areas, out-of-hospital maternity centers offer an alternative to hospital delivery for low-risk pregnancies.

HOME DELIVERY

It is ironic that at a time when U.S. hospitals are doing everything possible to change their blighted image as impersonal birth machines run on arbitrary rules and outmoded regulations, some prospective parents are bypassing hospitals and delivering their own babies in their homes—and they may be the start of a major trend.

This seemingly simple action—home delivery—has the traditional medical world in an uproar. The leaders of ACOG and many of its members across the nation consider home delivery extremely dangerous, akin to child abuse because of the risk it poses. They argue that no one knows when an obstetrical emergency will occur. They also bitterly oppose home birth attended by a lay midwife, a person with no formal training or certification. To document its case ACOG has collected data from many states showing greater risks to babies born out of hospital.

If you are contemplating a home delivery—and this *is* a serious matter—you should know that medical proponents of home delivery say that not all home deliveries pose equal risks. Dr. Lewis B. Mehl, M.D., of Berkeley, California, is an officer of a division of the National Association of Parents and Professionals for Safe Alternatives in Childbirth, a group based in Chapel Hill, North Carolina. He has written, "Planned home delivery of medically screened women by trained, competent doctors or midwives is different from home delivery of unscreened women with untrained, unskilled attendants or no attendants." The message of a highly controversial and potentially dangerous issue for pregnant women at this point in history is this: Home delivery is considered very hazardous by almost all experts. Some view it as safe if a pregnant woman has had good, thorough prenatal care, is considered a low risk—and if she can get competent, trained help for delivery.

Never attempt a delivery at home without being sure that you can get to a good hospital fast in case of an emergency. In troubled childbirth, minutes count.

HOW DO YOU CHOOSE THE RIGHT CARE?

Between the many options—various kinds of doctors and nurse-midwives, and different levels of hospitals—how do you choose what is right for you and your baby? "Right" does not mean the most popular obstetrician in town or the newest hospital. In some communities, clinic patients can get treatment as fine as or finer than private patients.

Although the price tag of your obstetrical care doesn't always determine its quality, cost is a significant aspect. One woman we interviewed shopped on a comparative-price basis for the most reasonable physician in a forty-mile radius of her Midwestern home, and chose the least expensive. It has been conservatively estimated that the cost of carrying, delivering and caring for a new baby through its first year is some $3,600. Prenatal and child-care costs vary greatly according to the service chosen and the standard rate in a particular community. The following are examples only. A nurse-midwife can be a bargain: under $1,000 for total prenatal and postnatal care, delivery and a two-day hospital stay; or $350 to $500 for midwife services minus hospital costs. In California, an obstetrician can charge $900; in New York City, $750; in a small town in Pennsylvania, $475; in Chicago, $600; and in Boston, as much as $1,000, just for maternal care and vaginal delivery. Furthermore, labor-and-delivery-room fees, anesthesia, baby's board in the nursery and mother's hospital stay are all extra. If a woman has a cesarean section, which means a longer hospital stay for both mother and child and an operating-room fee, costs can zoom to more than $4,000.

If cost alone doesn't determine the quality of your care, what yardstick should you use? Your yardstick is you—who you are medically and emotionally. To find out who you are medically, you need a rough idea of whether you are a low or high risk. Don't be afraid of the word *risk*. It refers only to a possibility, not a certainty, that you may have problems. "Risk" is a useful designation because it can help you find the right care.

Once again: The vast majority of pregnancies are normal, with healthy, noisy results. Pregnancy risk factors come into the picture when a woman has a personal history of certain illnesses, a family history, known or suspected, of genetic disorders, or a past history of obstetrical difficulties. Other risks arise when a healthy woman, having a normal pregnancy, develops a complication of pregnancy, such as hypertension, which requires special attention, or when she is beset by a medical problem unrelated to pregnancy, which could mean trouble for a developing baby. Another risk category revolves around labor and delivery: A woman may deliver prematurely, and prematurity and low birth weight are great dangers to newborns. Or she may go into labor full-term after a normal pregnancy, when an emergency delivery situation develops.

Good prenatal care means that your health condition and risk factors are constantly being screened and monitored. What kind of care you should have—nurse-midwife, family physician, board-certified obstetrician-gynecologist, perinatologist—depends on your risk profile, which can change during pregnancy. A pregnant diabetic woman, a genuine medical problem, may be at risk, but the risks can be minimized under expert care.

The woman with the most options in selecting health care during pregnancy is the woman in the low-risk category. A low-risk woman should be able to choose the care she prefers, but a woman who suspects a problem or who has had obstetrical difficulty in the past should seek a board-certified obstetrician affiliated with a level-II or III hospital. If it seems likely that you will be a candidate for a cesarean section, you want to have the operation performed by specialists with experience. Please remember that if cost is a great factor, teaching hospitals have residents (some of whom may qualify as junior fellows of ACOG), and experts are always available. A clinic with a sliding pay scale at a teaching hospital can be a solution to some problems.

WHERE DO YOU FIT IN?

Do you belong in the low-risk category? If you are under thirty-five, free of chronic medical diseases—hypertension, cardiac problems, endocrine disorders, neurological problems, or metabolic diseases, such as diabetes—you probably do. It helps if your nutritional status has been good most of your life and if you haven't abused yourself with cigarettes, alcohol or drugs. In the initial screening for any problems, physicians and nurse-midwives ask about known or suspected genetic or familial diseases among your relatives and your baby's father's family. They want to know if you have had two or more abortions or any kind of uterine operation.

If your medical history includes past pregnancy with a wanted child, what was your experience? Did you have a premature baby, a low-birth-weight baby, or a very large baby? At the time of labor, was the baby in an abnormal position? Have you had a prior cesarean section? Did your other baby or babies need neonatal care? Were there birth defects? Have you had two or more miscarriages? Do you have any diagnosed abnormalities of the genital tract or cervix, the neckline opening of the womb? Did your mother ever take large doses of prenatal estrogen, particularly DES (diethylstilbestrol)? (If your mother took estrogens, particularly DES, when she was carrying you, some physicians think you may experience an increased risk of cervical incompetence, although others find no such effect.) Was there ever a medical reason for ending a prior pregnancy? Did you ever deliver a stillborn or experience neonatal loss?

If you can answer no to these obstetrical questions, you may be in the low-risk category.

In addition to learning where you stand medically as a pregnant woman, you should ask yourself who you are emotionally as an individual entering a complex health care system. Do you prefer a strong doctor-patient relationship? Do you feel safest where there is a lot of equipment? Do you want your doctor to provide all of your care? Will you feel neglected if a nurse-practitioner talks to you about nutrition? Do you want to use a nurse-midwife? Will you be hassled by your husband, your mother and mother-in-law? Are you absolutely opposed to "natural" childbirth and worried about being bullied into it?

Pregnant women find their health care in a variety of ways. One woman picked her obstetrician out of the telephone book because she liked his name; another spent days in the library checking the credentials of half the obstetricians in Boston. A group of women in a Chicago suburb used the same obstetrical team for their pregnancies, and they recommended the team to pregnant newcomers to the community, not because the obstetricians were good but because, "as bad as they are, we know what they are like and they use a good hospital."

ZEROING IN ON YOUR CHOICE

There are several basic ways to find candidates for your obstetrical care and dollars.

Research. Names can be obtained and credentials checked through the sources on pages 217–20.

Referral. Names and assessments can be obtained from your other physicians. (Since even a trusted family doctor may be loathe to "bad-mouth" a colleague, listen for non-positives, like "he seems well trained" or "I haven't heard anything bad.") Other good sources include childbirth educators as well as labor-and-delivery-room nurses, who see obstetricians in action. Women who have *recently* given birth are helpful, but remember that reactions to doctors vary. (Ask friends *why* they like a particular doctor and to cite specific virtues and faults.)

Rating. Once you have at least two or three possibilities, you owe it to yourself to find the time—and money—to make an appointment and discover all you can about a particular doctor, nurse, midwife or obstetrical team before making your choice.

It is a wise idea to make a list of questions—some of them testers to draw conversation and reaction—to try on a preliminary or first visit to a doctor. A list with points most important to you is best. Here is a sample:

Basics. What is your hospital affiliation and what does the hospital offer? What are the total fees? What are your office procedures? Are there hours when you are available by telephone? Is there a fee for telephone consultation?

Prenatal. What are your views about the work I do? Will it influence my pregnancy? What about travel? I want to jog during pregnancy: Is that all right? If not, why not?

Delivery. Do you permit fathers in the delivery room? If I want a drug-free delivery, will you sign orders so that unasked-for medication will not automatically be given to me? What types of drugs do you use? When? Why?

Under what conditions will you do a cesarean? Do you induce labor? Why? Do you always do an episiotomy? (This is an incision of the tissue between your vaginal opening and rectum to prevent tearing when the baby's head emerges. It is often routine and may be unnecessary.)

On a screening visit try to determine who really is responsible and "in charge" of the office. It may be the doctor's wife, an unlicensed receptionist dressed in a nurse's uniform, or a nurse-practitioner who has advanced training. Try to determine if staff is a help or a hindrance. Some untrained office personnel have a tendency to try to answer the doctor's questions for them. Many women find themselves confiding in an office nurse because it seems easier than speaking with a doctor. If you find yourself doing this, think it over and speak to the person most responsible for your health care.

In many ways, your first official visit for prenatal care may be the most important event until you give birth. This visit should be at least forty-five minutes long, and every aspect of your health—including rubella immunization and nutrition—should be discussed. Whether or not your doctor asks, this is a time to describe fully your work habits, concerns about genetic problems, plans for travel, stresses in your life, questions about sex. After this visit, your doctor will spend only a few minutes with you. (Nurse-midwives are different in this regard.) For healthy pregnant women, prenatal care is a matter of weight and blood-pressure check, urine and other laboratory tests (there are indications that a prenatal test for neural tube defects, AFP or alpha-fetoprotein, may soon be widely used), a measurement of the growth of the fetus and listening to the fetal heartbeat. However, office visits should always include time for your questions, particularly emotional or sexual matters important to you.

CHANGING DOCTORS DURING PREGNANCY

Sometimes the maternity care that you have selected doesn't work out. You may discover, for example, that the doctor who said in your first trimester that he was in favor of prepared childbirth and is aware that you have taken classes suddenly begins to say that women have a low threshold for pain, that most women need medication, and that he will order some for you because his patients are usually grateful for it. Or you may find that your doctor is cold and impersonal and uninterested when you want to talk about the upsetting mood swings some women can experience. Or he or she may turn out to be unreliable because of personal problems, such as drinking. If you are in doubt—switch doctors.

On the medical level, you may develop swelling ankles, or your blood pressure may go up. This can be symptomatic of toxemia of pregnancy, and if you are being treated by a family doctor, you might want a consultation with an obstetrical specialist. Any physician who refuses a request for a consultation is just plain wrong.

Many women don't like to be branded "neurotic" or "doctor shoppers," but since in the New Pregnancy it is just fine to be on the "lemon list," it is better to trust your instincts and find the care that makes you the most confident and comfortable. You will probably have to pay only for the care you have received. Beyond that, you don't owe your doctor anything. You owe yourself a good pregnancy and a healthy baby.

OBSTETRICAL ISSUES IMPORTANT TO YOU

There is considerable controversy in obstetrics concerning intervention and technology. Obviously, women have given birth throughout the ages without benefit of fetal heart monitors, ultrasound and other new medical techniques. Equally obvious is the point that we don't want to give up the genuine benefits of technology. But despite the fact that most births are normal and may require little intervention, trained medical professionals are ready to go into battle with all the weapons of modern obstetrics.

Physicians are trained to respond to emergency, and we expect them to. Social historians who have traced childbirth in America have noted that physicians replaced midwives because they had access to such instruments as forceps. A family present at a nineteenth-century birth may well have expected action from a doctor to justify his presence and fee. Physicians became even more powerful with the advent of drugs to relieve the pain of childbirth. However, a woman under general or spinal anesthesia could not deliver her child unaided; therefore, the physician was required not only to give the medication but to help in the delivery by the use of forceps. Furthermore, forcep deliveries often required an episiotomy. Thus, childbirth often became a medical process rather than a spontaneous natural event. Said Dr. G.W. McLeod of Miami,

Florida, at a meeting of the South Atlantic Association of Obstetricians and Gynecologists: "I cannot think of another specialty in which the physician spends four years in postgraduate training and then spends the majority of his working hours taking care of patients undergoing a normal physiologic process."

It is an obstetrician's responsibility to know about advanced techniques; that is the emphasis in their teaching and their interest. Unusual approaches, for example, are not their basic concern. This is shown in the experience of Dr. David A. Kliot, clinical assistant professor of obstetrics and gynecology of the State University of New York Downstate Medical Center, who is one of the few American obstetricians enthusiastic about the Leboyer method. This is a way of greeting the newborn in a dimly lit room, where the baby is immediately given a massage and a bath. Because Dr. Kliot is at a teaching hospital, he opens his delivery room to obstetrical residents to witness this kind of delivery, which originated in France. Dr. Kliot explained, "Only a very, very few ever come. But when I do a forceps delivery, they really show up." What those residents are doing with their limited time is, however, very realistic. They are being trained for emergencies; they have to know equipment; it has to be part of their makeup to be aggressive when it comes to saving lives.

"There is no question that the welfare of their patients has always been the deep concern of American physicians, nurse-midwives and nurses," writes Doris Haire, consumer advocate and member of major committees of the National Institutes of Health, the U.S. Food and Drug Administration, and the American Public Health Association. "The unphysiological practices which have become so much a part of American obstetric care—to the point where such practices have been generally accepted as normal accompaniments of birth—appear to have gradually built up as a result of social customs and cultural patterning."

Some obstetric practices are questionable—and we will spotlight a few of them—but the cumulative effects can be dangerous. For example, if oxytocin is used to induce labor, contractions may be more rapid and strong. Even a woman trained in methods of prepared childbirth may have trouble dealing with pain and keeping control; she may require drugs, a forceps delivery and episiotomy. This sequence isn't bad if there is a genuine need to induce labor. Sometimes there is not.

It is difficult to sift the truth from all the shouting about obstetrical practices. This much is clear: An across-the-board condemnation of technology and intervention is as dangerous as unnecessary techniques. Some of the machinery, practices and attitudes of physicians are necessary. There are times when a physician has to be the judge of what is safe, proper and essential to save lives. Unfortunately, some physicians tend to state their case in a frightening and threatening way. If you have chosen your medical team with care and have built up an open relationship based on honesty, bullying shouldn't occur.

Most opponents of intervention and technology agree that special help is needed in some instances. In general, they object to routine application of certain procedures, some of which are still being questioned by the scientific community and government agencies. Here are some specifics.

Fetal Heart Monitoring

Fetal heart monitoring is a way of checking the condition of a baby in the womb by placing an external monitor on the mother's belly or an electrode on the baby's scalp while it is still in the womb. (This requires a natural or clinical rupturing of the amniotic sac.) It was developed to warn about high-risk deliveries, and it is a must when induced labor brings on contractions that are severe and rapid and may cause fetal distress. There are many genuine reasons why monitoring is used—for the woman with a high-risk health history; for the woman bearing twins; for a woman with vaginal bleeding—and there is documentation for the value of the technique. But, there are many indications that fetal monitoring is or very soon will be routine for almost all women hospitalized in labor. The need for routine monitoring of low-risk births is seriously questioned and far from certain.

A number of commentators and some studies have

shown that these machines are only as good as the professionals reading them. An error in interpreting certain early-model fetal monitors could lead to a needless emergency cesarean. As for the fetal monitor itself, former FDA Commissioner Dr. Donald Kennedy told a Senate health subcommittee in April 1978 that fetal monitoring "is not known to be without risk."

Presently there is a large educational effort aimed at professionals to teach monitoring and to encourage adherence to standards of interpretation. "With increasing evidence of the benefits derived from this technique, the concept of monitoring all patients is gaining support," says ACOG.

There is a certain irony that at a time when homelike birthing rooms with flowered wallpaper, regular beds, rocking chairs and soft lights are gaining popularity, there is a nationwide drive to hook every laboring woman up to a fetal monitor to the tune of $400 million extra each year. While the battle over fetal monitors goes on, it is useful to note a study done by Dr. Richard L. Cohen, professor and chief of child psychiatry at the University of Pittsburgh School of Medicine. Dr. Cohen studied behavioral and developmental problems in children whose mothers underwent fetal monitoring. It is Dr. Cohen's thesis that the mother's negative perception of the monitor may influence the early moments of family formation. The topic of fetal monitoring was introduced not by the interviewers in Dr. Cohen's study, but by the women questioned. Noting the importance of counseling all prospective parents about monitoring—since monitoring may need to be done in case of emergency even if it is refused for routine labor—Dr. Cohen told a meeting of the American Academy of Child Psychiatry that "particular attention should be paid to fantasies that portray the monitor as damaging the fetus or the mother, or in any way detracting from maternal participation in labor and delivery."

Ultrasound

Another technological advance under use but still open to question is diagnostic ultrasound, a technique using sound waves, not X-ray, that can detect a fetus even in the first trimester, show its development and be used as a form of monitoring. Fetal age is a very important fact to determine for good prenatal care and delivery, and ultrasound can help. The technique can also detect abnormal pregnancies and fetal abnormalities—for example heart defects. Dr. Kennedy reported in 1978 that "a prudent public health policy calls for judicious use of ultrasound where the expected benefits clearly outweigh the risks." In a patient education leaflet ACOG stated ". . . since this is a relatively new procedure it cannot be said with 100 percent certainty that it is completely safe."

Meanwhile, some obstetricians are now buying ultrasound equipment for their offices. But before have a "sonogram," you should discuss with your health team why it is required in your case. There are times when benefits outweigh risks and thus far no major dangers have been documented.

X-Rays

As a pregnant woman, you are probably aware that you should avoid all unnecessary radiation, especially to your abdomen, pelvis and back. X-rays pose risk of birth defects and other problems. And though you should always question the advisibility of having a diagnostic X-ray during pregnancy, there are times when the benefit outweighs the risk. For example, if you break a limb, X-rays may be very necessary.

Late in your pregnancy or during labor your medical team might need a pelvic X-ray to estimate pelvic and/or fetal size and to determine the safest means of delivery. This is a legitimate diagnostic procedure from which you can benefit. At one time, and perhaps today in some areas of the nation, it was common practice to order a series of pelvic films in the ninth month. Since there are other means of diagnosis (ultrasound, for instance) you should question this practice.

Cesareans and Malpractice

Another trend in modern obstetrics is the escalating rate of cesarean section which is of major concern. Once, this was an operation to be performed only out of dire necessity because of the danger of infection. However, better techniques, antibiotics and good nursing care have made a difference, and today obstetricians perform cesareans frequently, even when the matter is debatable, as in the case of a breech delivery.

Malpractice insurance cost and the threat of suits worry every physician practicing obstetrics—of the top twelve medical specialties sued most often, obstetrics is number three. You may be surprised to know that your obstetrician is liable for damages until your child is twenty-three. And in 1978, the St. Paul Fire and Marine Insurance Company, one of the largest carriers of professional liability insurance, reported that the number of obstetrician-gynecologists involved in malpractice disputes is growing. ACOG has had to devise malpractice insurance for its Fellows. Liability and the trend towards litigation may make your physician order many tests and take very conservative action on medical matters. This is called defensive medicine. If there are doubts, he or she may be more likely to perform a cesarean.

If you do deliver by cesarean section for whatever reason (and there are some very good reasons), you should know that in some communities there are self-help groups (that you can find through childbirth educators) composed of people who have gone through the cesarean experience and can offer valuable insights. If you have time to think about it before a cesarean, you may want to request a spinal or epidural anesthesia so that you may see and touch your new baby seconds after birth. This arrangement is not always permitted, so you will have to ask. If you are going to have a planned cesarean or if there is time to make a request, you may want to ask if your husband can be present. Although often a great benefit because it means a healthy baby, a cesarean birth is a different physical and emotional experience from a natural birth. Each pregnant woman should know about cesarean birth, because there is always the possibility that it might be necessary. As for the rule, "Once a cesarean always a cesarean," if the prior delivery was necessitated by a complication that is unlikely to recur, a woman may be allowed a "trial of labor" for her next delivery. There is a definite trend towards vaginal delivery after prior cesarean although individual obstetricians may have fixed opinions. However, there is documentation for the rationale of at least trying vaginal birth—a study of 500 pregnant women reported in a major ACOG journal showed that almost half could deliver vaginally with safety despite a prior cesarean.

Induced Labor

There are many reasons for a physician to set labor in motion, which he or she does by opening the membrane of the amniotic sac, by intravenous infusion of oxytocin, or by a combination of the two techniques. If induction is done by drugs, surveillance of mother and child through monitors and other means should be done. It may be absolutely necessary to induce labor if there is suspected fetal distress or if the membranes have ruptured prematurely and natural labor hasn't begun, raising the risk of infection. Induced labor is more difficult for the mother to control, and the hormones used can cause complications. But the power to induce labor is a rather neat trick in the obstetrical world's medical bag. It allows a doctor who is contemplating a vacation to deliver babies who are near term before he leaves town. A woman who wants to attend a wedding and whose baby is dawdling in the womb may also badger her doctor into inducing labor. The problem is premature babies. A baby born too soon can often run into serious difficulties. Usually ACOG is very neutral and detached in its technical bulletins to members on this matter. However, in a 1978 bulletin on induced labor the nation's obstetricians were warned not to be the causes of premature birth.

DEALING WITH YOUR DOCTOR

Making the medical system work for you and your baby requires that you know the facts about obstetrical options and the current issues. It also means that you must be willing to deal with the medical world with strength and confidence. As women shared their pregnancy experiences for this book it became obvious that a crucial topic was the pregnant woman's relationship with her physician. With eagerness and some relief, pregnant women wanted to talk about their doctors, how they were being treated, what was right, what was wrong. Many of their feelings may be your feelings.

Many women interviewed were angry and disillusioned. They were disappointed in themselves for not being able to command the kind of treatment and respect that they felt that they deserved. Some of these pregnant women were highly esteemed professionals—including physicians and a college dean—and some were physicians' wives and daughters.

From their experiences, from research and commentary— much of it done by women—we can help explain why you may have trouble dealing with the medical world. We will explain some of the influences that may be shaping your attitudes and affecting the way you are treated. There are ways to make this aspect of your pregnancy better.

There are two factors that influence women's dealings with the medical world. The first is the male medical profession's essentially negative view of women and their health. It is a view that shows signs of changing, but it results in the humiliating way women are sometimes treated, which gives them subtle messages about their inferiority and powerlessness, and increases both. The second is women's unquestioning acceptance of medical authority.

THE MEDICAL VIEW OF WOMEN

Traditionally, women have not been treated as substantial human beings by their male doctors. Obstetrics and gynecology in particular, being medical specialties practiced by men on women, often expose women to humiliation. Any patient, male or female, is usually in an inferior position, but in the eyes of the medical world there is something suspect about female complaints and the female body.

Since ancient times, woman's womb has been associated with hysteria—the Greek *hystera* was the word for uterus. The ancients thought the womb was capable of traveling through the body, causing havoc and illness unless occupied by pregnancy. In the nineteenth century, thanks to the invention of the speculum by an American, J. Marion Sims, gynecologists first saw the vagina, cervix and discharges from the uterus. As Dr. John Haller, associate professor of history at the University of Indiana Northwest has noted, women's health and behavior became comprehensible. "Doctors began attributing almost all of women's illnesses to inflammation or ulceration of the cervix . . . the theory held for some twenty years and was blamed for nausea, uterine inertia, sexual dysfunction, disorders of the liver and kidneys, hysterical symptoms . . ."

That was the nineteenth century. In the twentieth, Gena Corea, the author of *The Hidden Malpractice*, has observed, "Consider what gynecology books written by men taught me about women: that her hormonal system makes her utterly unlike men in her ambitions and abilities; that menstrual pain often merely reflects her psychological shortcomings; that she tends to invent symptoms so physicians must not take her complaints too literally; that she becomes repulsive at menopause. In a 1966 book, one gynecologist referred to the menopausal woman as 'living decay'; that her sex drive is inferior to man's and relatively unimportant."

While there are many indications that those messages have been mostly rewritten for medical students, they are still in the minds of some graduates now practicing obstetrics. Attitudinal change in the medical world is slow.

Dr. Mary Howell, M.D., Ph.D., of Harvard University, wrote in 1974, "It is widely taught, both explicitly and implicitly, that women patients (when they receive notice at all) have uninteresting illnesses, are unreliable historians, and are beset by such emotionality that their symptoms are unlikely to reflect 'real disease.' "

Pregnant women have gotten a lot of clear messages about what the medical profession thinks of them, and this may help explain why some women feel and act as if in the presence of a superior force. In 1968, a book entitled *The World of a Gynecologist* noted that ". . . if he [the gynecologist] is kind, then his kindness and concern for his patient may provide her with a glimpse of God's image."

HOW FEMALE PATIENTS ARE TREATED

It is worth spelling out some of the annoying aspects of medical care that clearly reflect what the medical world thinks of women and the value it places on women's time. Most of these annoyances take place in your physician's office; in fact, one perceptive woman called office visits "rituals of humiliation." These rituals can be impossibly long waits in a doctor's office; rushed examinations; impersonality; condescension; a subtle emphasis on the almost magical power of the physician. One woman we spoke to said her doctor asked her, when she came for a postnatal checkup, if he or his partner had delivered her baby. Another woman, a high school biology teacher, said her doctor kept referring to ovulation as "making an egg, as if no woman could understand so complicated a word as 'ovulation.' "

As for waits in doctors' offices, in a physician profile study done by the University of Southern California, questioning of a random sample of 879 obstetrician-gynecologists across the nation showed that an average of 9.8 minutes is spent on each patient encounter, in contrast to the long time spent in the waiting room before the doctor sees the patient. This means that a prenatal office visit may be even shorter than 9.8 minutes, because the average figure was compiled from time spent as well on hospital visits, medical procedures, surgery and telephone calls. In obstetrics time is money, and when it comes to waiting for care, woman's time has a low value.

The idea that the medical world has special, almost magical power exists everywhere. Many women—some because of their mates, some because of birth-control pills, some because of physical or emotional problems—have difficulty in conceiving, and must endure a series of rigorous and unpleasant fertility tests during a time of great emotional strain. We interviewed one woman who was having difficulty conceiving who told us that while she was talking to her gynecologist, his partner came in and said, "Don't worry, *we'll* get you pregnant." Another woman, whose fertility specialist was also her obstetrician, said that he suggested, only half-joking, that she name the baby after him.

Many women who have not had conception difficulties believe that their physicians are responsible for childbirth, and they express this belief by thanking doctors for their babies. Social worker Patsy Turrini of the Mothers' Center, Long Island, New York, has noted that this mistaken idea is often prompted by from the fact that it is the doctor who confirms that there is indeed a baby in the womb when he first hears the fetal heartbeat. Until that moment when the doctor applies the stethoscope to the womb or a Doppler sounding device, which can confirm life at nine weeks, a woman can only really know that she is pregnant because of a test, a weight gain, swollen breasts, nausea, missed periods. Thus some women tend to believe the physician is critical to the life and death of the baby. During labor the doctor may even seem godlike.

In addition to attributing mythical qualities to them, some women become overly dependent on their doctors. Medicine's traditional view of women is reinforced by some women's submissiveness and passivity. This is doctor dependence, and most pregnant women have it to some degree. But even if you are very much in control of your medical care during pregnancy and have a fine, mutually respectful relationship with your physician or nurse-midwife, it is natural to feel a loss when, after nine months of involvement, the relationship cuts off abruptly with the postpartum checkup.

If pregnant women are excessively doctor dependent, they may transfer this dependency after pregnancy to their child's pediatrician, or may return to their obstetrician-gynecologist with some vague complaints. Also when pregnant women depend on their doctor too much, they may be totally unable to criticize or change doctors if the care is unsatisfactory. Many women complain privately but feel unable to do anything.

Whether women need to believe in the authority of doctors or whether they have been trained by society and manipulated by doctors to give over authority to a medical force is an unsettled question. What is documented is that doctor dependence exists to an alarming degree in pregnancy. So be wary.

AND NOW—FOR THE BRIGHT SIDE!

There has been so *very* much to enrage women about the male medical profession "in charge" of the female body that it is emotionally satisfying and intellectually easy to list grievances. But there has been rapid, even extraordinary change, with the promise of more to come in the immediate future. To cling to anger rather than to seek out the new and good is a terrific waste of energy—particularly when one is pregnant.

"People ask me, 'What are you going to do about your profession?' " comments Dr. Marcia Storch, an assistant clinical professor at the Columbia University College of Physicians and Surgeons. "I say, 'Thank you very much, my profession is doing fine.' Where change really begins—in clinics, medical schools, textbooks and meetings—the teaching today stresses the importance of making more services and information and more self-responsibility and choices available to women."

This comment comes from a physician who is deeply concerned with women's rights, and who began her own career when the attitude of her male colleagues was, that if a woman could do it, it wasn't worth doing.

"This is a happy field, not one in which you are dealing mainly with cancer or coronaries," says Dr. Ivan Strausz, a Manhattan obstetrician-gynecologist who has helped train female residents in the specialty. "I have worked in several different kinds of communities, and I have seen a gradual change from women who wanted to be totally drugged to women who are bright enough and care enough to deliver their babies in the most natural way possible."

Other signs of progress: The American College of Obstetricians and Gynecologists, which assiduously avoids all save medical politics, has endorsed the proposed equal rights amendment; *Our Bodies, Ourselves,* the "bible" of the women's self-help movement, is a national bestseller;

and physicians are beginning to respond to the New Pregnancy and to show a concern for women's occupations, stresses and requests to be treated well.

Further evidence of this change: Dr. Ronald J. Bolognese, director, Section on Perinatology, Pennsylvania Hospital in Philadelphia, has a psychological counselor as a co-worker to help women cope with the emotional demands of pregnancy. This is an innovation indeed. In Hempstead, New York, and elsewhere mothers or parenting centers offer a program of emotional and practical support for pregnant women and new mothers. Volunteers from the Hempstead center travel to local hospitals to inform professionals of maternal needs. In Boston, healthy women allow medical students to practice pelvic examinations on them so that they can have a few minutes to explain how women should be treated as patients. In San Francisco, a storefront health group teaches women how to do diagnostic tests and use the stethoscope so that they can monitor their baby's heartbeat. In the Midwest, there is a strong prepared-childbirth movement.

Basic change in the medical world begins on the educational level. In 1975 a totally different kind of textbook, *Obstetrics and Gynecology: The Health Care of Women,* was published. This 1,163-page volume by many authors opens with "The Physician's Responsibility," in which Dr. James A. Merrill, professor and head of gynecology-obstetrics at the University of Oklahoma, states, "The women's health movement has focused attention upon what some women consider to be demeaning in gynecological care. This requires an attitudinal change on the part of physicians if they are to keep abreast of the changes that are occurring rapidly in our society."

In an interview, the book's senior author, Dr. Seymour L. Romney, professor of obstetrics and gynecology at New York's Albert Einstein College of Medicine, explained, "We tried to create a book that would be nontraditional and recognize change. We took a comprehensive approach to women's health. We felt that women have many things to do in life besides having babies." In an early chapter of the book, four social scientists—three of them women—present the facts about the new status of women, their special problems and angers. After listing problem areas similar to the ones we have discussed, the book notes, "Overall, these criticisms may or may not be representative, *but they represent anguish of a sort men rarely experience.*"

Some of the message of the women's health movement has been heard and heeded.

TAKING CONTROL

It is now up to you to reap some of the benefits of the change that has been achieved thus far. You *can* retune yourself.

- At your first prenatal visit you can explain in a firm, clear way what your expectations for maternal care are.

- You can ask to be addressed by your full name or title, not your first name, unless you call your physician by his or her first name.

- You can ask to speak to your physician in his or her office when you are dressed and more in command of yourself than when you are a patient in a paper robe.

- If you want more time from your physician, offer to pay for it to show that you are serious and fair.

- Demand the true facts about your health.

- If you want a consultation, you can be more firm if you have researched the problem and can be specific about why you want added expertise.

- Always have written questions in hand when you see your physician, because it is easy to forget things under the stress of a quick examination; take notes of answers for your own clarity and reference; always question what is being done— why do I need this test?

- Never act apologetic about asking a physician anything—don't create a situation that puts you on the defensive.

- Never allow a physician to "yell" at you or treat you abusively.

- If an answering service, office nurse or relief physician (who may work weekends) is rude or slow or a problem, tell your doctor and be specific.

- Encourage your husband to meet your doctor and keep your husband informed of your treatment, so that if you want to change doctors you will have emotional support.

- If you encounter an "obstetrical lemon," let your friends know. You may be embarrassed that you had a bad experience, but if you are willing to admit it, you can help others and free your anger.

Times are changing. As more women live the New Pregnancy and participate in their medical care, the obstetrical world will have to respond. Some obstetricians may even like the change. Dr. Charles Flowers of the University of Alabama told his peers at an annual ACOG clinical meeting, "I recently had an interesting experience of a patient who wanted to have a home delivery and her husband was afraid for her to have one. She came in with a single-spaced, two-page list of demands. I sat down with her and sort of felt like a management-labor negotiator going over each point with her. In the end I was glad I did because we were able to compromise on several of these points."

After pregnancy and delivery, one woman we interviewed said, "I had very positive experiences. You hear so many horror stories—and I had read them too—that I was prepared to put up with a lot, and I *never* expected an enlightened progressive attitude. In the past gynecologists had kind of patted me on the head and said the not-to-worry kind of thing. But my obstetricians never did. They dealt with me as an adult, as a person who could understand complex situations. They presented the options and left the decision to me. I appreciated that very much, and as a result I felt very free about asking questions. Of course, I worked and traveled. They all told me, 'You're not sick, keep on doing what you are doing.'

"My husband and I took childbirth education classes; we used a combination labor-and-delivery room. My husband was there all the time. We had zero interference. It was really our show all the way!"

3

SPORTS

"I was a little shaky the first few steps, but that was because I hadn't been on skates for a while and I was eight months pregnant at the time. It only took me a few times around the rink and I really felt good."

> 1976 Olympic medalist Sheila Young

"They said it wasn't fair bowling two against one, but that was the only criticism I received from my competitors."

> Betty Morris, championship bowler who won her first tournament when she was six months pregnant

"Most physicians are not familiar with female athletes, and in particular female fencers. They have a vision of Errol Flynn jumping over stair railings—and it really isn't that way at all."

> Jan Romary, ten times a women's national fencing champion

"There is more emphasis in people's minds today that pregnancy is not a state of disability, but rather that it is part of a normal lifestyle. It is not a time to retreat from the world, but to keep up one's activity and participation in it."

> Allan Ryan, M.D., editor, *The Physician and Sportsmedicine* magazine

Women in increasing numbers are swinging tennis rackets, swimming, running and participating in a variety of physical activities as never before—all part of the increased national awareness of physical fitness.

Whereas only a few years ago physical activity was equated with musty gymnasiums and oversized bloomers or gym suits, today it means fitness and good health. No longer are women who participate in sports activities labeled "jocks" or considered unfeminine. It is suddenly fashionable to be fit—and fitness has become an integral part of the active woman's life.

What happens, then, when you become pregnant? Do the same rules that applied when you were not pregnant apply now?

Physical activity *can* be part of your pregnancy. If you have regularly participated in a sport, then pregnancy alone is no reason to stop. There are precautions to take, however, and we will discuss these along with suggestions on how to accommodate your changing figure. We will also tell you how to provide for changes in balance, posture and pacing for your selected sport during the next nine months.

Not only has general information about the benefits of physical activity for the pregnant woman been largely unavailable, but until now there has been little information for women participating in any major sport. To fill this void, we went to the female pros in the various sports fields who had been pregnant to see how they worked it out and to ask what suggestions they could offer to you.

Because of their cooperation and enthusiasm we are able to offer you the first complete guide to sports participation for the pregnant woman.

GOOD FOR YOUR BODY, GOOD FOR YOUR MIND

When asked whether she thought sports participation during pregnancy is good for body and mind, horsewoman Sally Ike, member of the United States Equestrian Team at the 1968 Mexico City Olympics, said, "Absolutely."

Ike rode, jumped and showed horses throughout both of her pregnancies, and concluded that "if it is something you do regularly, you will be much better off. If you stop, then you are going to sit around twiddling your thumbs, wondering what you are going to do with your time. And then you get into head problems."

Tennis champion Margaret Court played throughout all three of her pregnancies. "My doctor is a great believer in exercise," she said. "Tennis is something I've done my whole life, and he felt it would be more harmful to stop doing something that I was used to. Playing the way I play, however, I had to make sure I didn't get carried away and do the things that I would do in a tournament. I didn't smash a lot, but rather played just for the exercise."

An active woman is a smart woman, and the Victorian notion that a woman must be shielded from physical and emotional stress just doesn't hold up in a modern pregnancy. Although each case is different and you should check with your doctor regarding your own personal situation, generally, the experts agree that the benefits of activity during pregnancy far outweigh any chance of injury. Dr. Dorothy V. Harris, director of the Center for Women and Sports at Pennsylvania State University, summed up the benefits in two short sentences: "Pregnancy is a physiological function. When the body is in good shape everything functions better." According to Harris, statistics have shown that women who exercise have had easier and safer deliveries, fewer premature births, shorter labors and, quite possibly, healthier children.

In a survey of 800 Hungarian athletes, Dr. Gyula J. Erdelyi, now a practicing obstetrician-gynecologist in Cleveland, Ohio, found that menarche, menstruation and pregnancies were not adversely affected by vigorous training. Additional studies have demonstrated that exercise helps alleviate and oftentimes prevent lower back pain that accompanies pregnancy.

In an interview, Dr. Erdelyi talked about his work and its relationship to the woman who is active but not an athlete: "In a normal situation there should be no problem with any type of exercise. If the pregnancy is intact, if there is no bleeding, no cramping, then there is no harmful effect at all. There is, in fact, widespread knowledge that physical activity gives one not only better physical health, but emotional health as well."

A symposium sponsored by *The Physician and Sportsmedicine* magazine lends support to the belief in the benefits of exercise during pregnancy. Four prominent physicians, all active in the field of sportsmedicine, discussed pregnancy and sports participation. Among the conclusions the participants reached were:

● Athletes had fewer complications of pregnancy and delivery.

● There is no apparent evidence that female athletes have any difficulties in conceiving.

● The first stage of labor is shorter in athletes than in nonathletes.

● Many athletes perform better after giving birth to one or more children.

A study conducted by Dr. Evalyn Gendel, director of the Human Sexuality Program at the University of California, San Francisco Medical School, measured the relationship between the level of physical fitness and chronic complaints. Not surprisingly, the more fit the woman, the less physical complaints she had.

Take, as an example, a third-time pregnant woman who is also the women's track coach at a major Midwestern university. This woman said, "I've had a lot of trouble this time around and I'm convinced that it's because I haven't been as active as in my previous two pregnancies. In those I swam, rode my bike, lifted weights, and the pregnancies were so easy. This pregnancy, to be perfectly honest, has been a real bummer. You've got to stay active to feel good."

A few of the major benefits the average woman can expect from a regular program of exercise or sports activity during her pregnancy are an improved cardiovascular system, which promotes circulatory and respiratory fitness to help her get through the extra weight gain and delivery; greater endurance and fitness for labor and delivery; a sense of well-being and higher self-esteem, especially postpartum, when the "mother machine" has completed her duties.

Boston surgeon, 1956 Olympic figure-skating champion and mother of three, Tenley Albright offers the following comment on the postpregnancy benefits of exercise: "It's much easier to do whatever you want afterward when you have stomach muscles that will snap back. That's why physical activity is an advantage rather than a disadvantage."

A leading West Coast sportsmedicine specialist said, "There is no reason that a healthy young woman should not benefit from physical activity as long as her pregnancy is healthy and her physician has no objections."

But there are still many women who fear that their baby will "jiggle loose" or that they will suffer a miscarriage if they participate in physical activity. Is there any basis for these fears?

A good rule to follow before any physical activity program is begun is to check with your physician or medical support team. Ask whether there are any physical conditions in your own pregnancy that might jeopardize the fetus. There *are* instances, depending on your previous history and individual case, where your physician might recommend a more limited schedule, especially during the first two or three months, when the dangers of disturbing the pregnancy are greatest.

In early pregnancy your body is making the most adjustments and may, in fact, spontaneously abort. But this is nature's way of saying that something is wrong, and early miscarriage is now known to be often caused by the death of a defective ovum or fetus. Today it is generally accepted by medical science that physical activity in itself is not directly the cause of miscarriage.

Dr. Carl Javert, in his book *Spontaneous and Habitual Abortion,* described his study of 2,000 cases of miscarriage. In his original study he found that out of all these cases of miscarriage, only seven occurred after the women had been in some kind of physical danger. Five of the women had fallen; two had been in minor car accidents. And further examination showed that in every case there was some additional problem with the developing fetus. Subsequent follow-up studies substantiated Javert's original research.

One condition in which physical activity is *not* recommended is cervical incompetence. This means that the cervix is either dilated or weakened, and can cause a second-trimester miscarriage. In most instances, the cervix will be stitched to prevent early opening and physical activity will be forbidden. Your physician or medical support team will tell you if you have this condition.

Other conditions where physical activity may not be recommended is (1) toxemia, where a woman has two of the following symptoms: albumin in the urine, high blood pressure and/or edema (swelling); or (2) a placenta previa, in which the placenta is either completely or partially covering the opening to the cervix. In instances where these symptoms exist, the physician or medical support person should be aware of them and discuss the individual situation accordingly.

In general, however, in a normal situation physical activity is beneficial, and the woman who participates in sports is unlikely to abide by the rules her mother and older sister lived by years ago. Take, for example, the advice that *Good Housekeeping* magazine was offering its readers in 1936: "You must accept the fact that as far as you are concerned, sports for the time being are out. You can take sunbaths; swim in still water, not surfs, as long as your doctor allows; work in the garden; do the usual office and light housework."

If All-American bowler Betty Morris had followed this advice, she never would have won her first title—when she was six months pregnant. When asked whether she had any qualms about bowling while pregnant, Morris said, "A few, but not enough to stop me from bowling. I never changed anything, I never tried to baby myself. And when it became uncomfortable for me to bowl, I stopped—that was at about seven and a half months."

CONVENTIONAL WISDOM

Conventional wisdom, however, is still very strong, causing many women to be uncertain whether to continue their sports participation during their pregnancies. This type of wisdom, however, is often based on ignorance, misconception and old wives' tales.

Tenley Albright told us, "I have been involved with many patients in early pregnancy, especially if they have fertility problems and require surgery. One thing that has always surprised me is that they feel they have to stop being active." When asked to what she attributed this, Albright said, "I think we are apt to think what we are expected to think or what we have been brought up to think."

Are there logical reasons for the conventional wisdom that makes many women uncertain whether they should continue their activity during their pregnancy and that often makes physicians counsel against activity? Let's examine a few.

The lack of interest by women in sports activity. It has been only within the past decade that women have begun to participate in sports in large numbers, and, therefore, there was no need until now to bring up any questions relating to sports and pregnancy.

Discomfort experienced by many women in early pregnancy. Dr. Albright explained that in the first few weeks of pregnancy many women experience a degree of discomfort, perhaps nausea or morning sickness. Although the discomfort ceases, she said, many women believe that the entire pregnancy is going to be this way—and by then, they have ceased an active routine.

Lack of approval by peers and parents. Many times one's actions are determined by one's relatives or peers, and many women interviewed stated that they received numerous comments and questions about their activity from men and women, usually, but not always, from an older generation.

One strong-minded tennis player, in discussing how she countered her husband's concern, said, "He finally realized that this was something I was going to do whether or not he approved." Another active woman who played racquetball through most of her pregnancy felt that "as women keep playing sports, more men and women will become more educated about it. It is the woman's choice. It is not going to hurt her."

Lack of knowledge by obstetricians about fitness and the benefits of exercise. "Unfortunately, we in the medical field have treated pregnancy as a disease, which it isn't," Dr. Evalyn Gendel said. Penn State's Harris added, "It depends on the physician and his awareness and his own sports activity, but you can generalize that most don't have a good understanding of physiology and exercise."

Dr. Ralph Hale, an obstetrician and women's team physician at the University of Hawaii, said that "most physicians have been doing crisis-oriented care and have not been concerned with preventive care." When asked to what he attributed the changing attitudes of physicians, Hale said, "Now there is no longer a negative view. Previously there was a negative attitude because of the lack of information. Nobody really knew, so they just assumed that activity was bad for you. We are only now beginning to see that this isn't so."

The fear of malpractice suits. One other explanation for the lack of physician support for sports activity during pregnancy was offered by Dr. Rudolph Dressendorfer, an exercise physiologist at the University of California at Davis, who recently completed a two-year study on the effects of exercise on a pregnant woman. He noted that physicians have been reluctant to go out on a limb because of the fear of malpractice. There are currently no guidelines for the obstetrical establishment to follow when recommending an exercise program to a healthy woman with a normal pregnancy. (Such guidelines currently exist for cardiac patients or patients with muscular difficulties.) Dr. Dressendorfer thinks that if guidelines existed the obstetrician could check the guidelines and follow them accordingly.

"A physician has to be very careful today," he continued. "He must know his patient. The major concern, of course, regards the safety of exercise for the mother and the fetus. A researcher or a physiologist is not responsible for malpractice. They can conduct the research and perform the studies, but it is up to the physician to interpret the findings."

Dr. Clayton Thomas, vice-president and medical affairs director of Tampax, Incorporated, summed up the question of participation in sports during pregnancy during *The Physician and Sportsmedicine* magazine symposium: "This should be an individual matter. In the present time, we tend to believe that the pregnant woman should be protected from strenuous athletics. This attitude is inconsistent with what many woman have found to be possible."

The three pregnant women who won gold medals at the 1956 Melbourne Olympics would agree, as would Margaret Court and Evonne Goolagong, who continued to play noncompetitive tennis during their pregnancies; Cathy Rigby, who taught gymnastics during her pregnancy; and Juno Irwin, who won a bronze medal in diving competition at the 1952 Olympics when she was three months pregnant.

PRECAUTIONS TO TAKE

One thing that virtually everyone agrees with—and this includes physicians, sportsmedicine specialists, women athletes and pregnant women themselves—is that pregnancy is probably not a good time to begin an exercise program. A twenty-four-year-old swimmer, mother of two and member of the 1968 Olympic team said, "It's hard when you start anything new. And because of the tiredness most women experience during their pregnancy, beginning any sports activity at this time would be difficult."

So be cautious and realistic, and ask yourself the following question: What was your fitness level before you became pregnant? If you were active before, then you can try to maintain your fitness level as much as possible during pregnancy.

Dr. Ralph Hale tells his patients who are used to activity to continue their normal schedules through the first six months. Then they will probably begin to experience some tiredness because of the physical demands of the body during the last trimester of the pregnancy, and they should probably slow down a bit.

As far as precautions regarding a blow to the uterus, with ordinary activity there is virtually no chance of affecting the uterus. Dr. Harris illustrates this: "Think of the fetus as an egg floating in a dish of water. It can't break. The uterus is the same thing. It is very well protected."

Activity during pregnancy varies from sport to sport and from person to person, explains Dr. Allan Ryan, editor of *The Physician and Sportsmedicine* magazine: "If you are participating in a vigorous sort of activity, don't do anything you are not used to doing. When you are exercising, note if there is a significant difference in the way you feel either during or immediately after participation. If there is a difference, check with your physician."

Gretchen Spruance, five times women's national squash champion, who was twenty-seven when she had her son Jake, suggested, "Listen to your body. Let your body tell you what is going on. Do as much as you feel capable of doing as long as you listen to the warning signals. If you are dying to play, then play, but listen to your body when it tells you to stop."

In other words, train but don't strain.

PHYSICAL ACTIVITY AND YOUR CHANGING BODY

The major change many pregnant women experience is largely due to an alteration in the center of gravity—which becomes lower because of the gain in weight and the change in circumference. If you are active, however, you probably won't notice how your continually changing body affects your fitness activity, because the changes in your body will happen gradually.

A twenty-eight-year-old mother of two who played tennis, ran and swam throughout her pregnancies said that the only difference she noticed in her tennis game was her backhand: "I just couldn't get my right arm around my belly. I could still hit a fairly accurate backhand, but I didn't have my total strength."

Another tennis player, who taught up to the day she delivered, said that sometimes she would stretch to get a ball, and "my stomach would hit my knee."

There is also a little-known change that can occur during the latter months of pregnancy and can be uncomfortable. Normally, the two pubic bones are attached where they meet in the lower front area. During pregnancy this junction becomes softened, and the bones may even separate. This may cause discomfort if one moves either leg up or down as much as one inch. Ask your physician or health support person, but it is probably best to stop your activity if this should occur.

Balance

Along with the physical changes of the body during pregnancy, there will be some adjustments regarding balance during the nine-month period. These adjustments, also due to changes in the center of gravity, are subtle.

Cathy Rigby, world champion gymnast, who competed in the 1968 and 1972 Olympics and was the fifth highest ranking female gymnast in the world when she retired, taught gymnastics during her pregnancy. She noticed a change in balance affected her gymnastic activity: "When I did handstands, I noticed I kept falling back down because my balance was so different and I had to compensate for the added weight."

Tennis player Margaret Court said that she, too, had problems with coordination at the beginning of her pregnancies, but within the first few months her balance was reestablished. Squash champion Gretchen Spruance noticed that she had to stand with her feet farther apart as she got farther along in her pregnancy in order to maintain her balance. And All-American bowler Cheryl Robinson, who competed in tournaments until her fifth month, said her balance improved during her pregnancy. With the added weight, she said, she tended to approach the line slower and release the ball with a great deal more accuracy.

Posture

Better muscle tone equals better posture. If you are fit you will probably have better muscle tone, which will aid in eliminating one of pregnancy's major complaints— backaches.

Backaches occur largely as a result of strain on the back muscles emanating from the spine. If you practice good posture, there is likely to be less strain on these muscles and thus less backache.

Pacing

Once again, there is virtual agreement on the subject of pacing. Pace yourself on the basis of how you feel. Take a relaxed attitude and don't push yourself. Realize that physiological changes are occurring and you must adjust to these changes. If the exercise is too much, then stop.

Nina Kuscsik, R.N., American women's record holder in the fifty-mile run and mother of three, said, "Each person should be an experiment of one and do what is best for that individual person. Don't let yourself get worn down, because if you do, no one wins. The baby will take what it needs and the mother will suffer."

"Rest is also very important," Sheila Young says. "If I was active for a period of time, I would make sure I had a good meal and rested for a while."

Gretchen Spruance reiterated, "Let your body tell you when to stop. I remember seeing stars a few times, and obviously I had moved too quickly. I then just had to slow down and not make such a great effort."

Clothing

There is currently a wide variety of attractive sports clothing available for the pregnant woman, including tennis dresses, running shorts and bathing suits. Wear what is most comfortable for you.

If your legs are very tired from your activity and the temperature is not overly hot, you may want to wear support stockings to relieve some of the discomfort you may experience.

You may also have to accommodate your enlarged breasts with a support bra. Several women athletes noted that a bra with a wider band provided better support for their breasts during their activities.

Activity for the Nonactive Woman

Since there is general agreement that pregnancy is not a good time to begin a formal exercise program, what can the nonactive woman do if she wants to exercise? First, ask your physician, but there is no reason, if you are healthy and the pregnancy is normal, that a program of walking and light jogging cannot be beneficial.

The late Dr. John L. Marshall, who was director of sportsmedicine at New York's Hospital for Special Surgery, team physician for many professional teams, and trainer of Billie Jean King, Rosie Casals and other pros, suggested practicing the basic abdominal strengthening exercises as a way of preparing the stomach muscles for childbirth and enabling the nonactive woman to have some degree of exercise.

In this exercise, somewhat like a modified sit-up, the knees should be bent with the feet remaining on the floor. With arms held forward, raise the shoulders off the floor and move the chest forward until the curved back comes halfway to the knees. Return to starting position very slowly, and repeat ten times daily, or until the onset of fatigue. (The Lamaze method of prepared childbirth also emphasizes a series of abdominal exercises designed to strengthen the stomach muscles.)

Injuries

Pregnancy is one time when the added stress of an athletic injury is certainly not desirable. It is probably wise, however, to consider possible injuries and anticipate alternatives for treatment.

Dr. Marshall, who was also co-chairman of the New York Medical Society's Committee on Medical Aspects of Sports, said that because women tend to be more loose-jointed than men, they are more susceptible to injuries involving the ligaments and joints. The most important factor to remember is not to lose control, but to do what you would normally do within your own ability.

Marshall said, "There are problems with regard to the treatment of surgical situations because of the surgical setting and the potential requirement for a general anesthetic. But we don't see this too often." He emphasizes that if a pregnant woman experiences a serious injury, she should try to avoid taking drugs and anti-inflammatory agents. Depending on the stage of the pregnancy, or the type and position of the injury, and on the future ramifications for the mother, the decision to have X-rays taken should be weighed with care. If X-rays are necessary, the uterus should be shielded with a lead apron. In addition, if an injury requires a cast, the cast may have to be replaced at some point during the healing process because of swelling that often occurs as a result of pregnancy.

GENERAL ADVICE FOR SPORTS PARTICIPATION

One of the major concerns of pregnant women who take part in sports is the amount of oxygen used by the mother and fetus. It is feared that if the mother uses up excess oxygen, not enough will go to the fetus, thus possibly damaging the baby.

Dr. Joan Ullyot, marathon runner, exercise physiologist, director of the Aerobics and Physiology Division of the Institute of Health Research in San Francisco, and mother of two, suggests the "talk test" as a guideline in determining whether or not you are using excess oxygen. If you can continue to talk easily while exercising, she says, then you are not overdoing it, not working at capacity and not using excess oxygen. Thus, both mother and fetus are assured of maintaining an adequate supply of oxygen.

Here then, are a few hints for each of the major sports in which women participate today.

TENNIS

"I wouldn't advise playing competitively," said Margaret Court. When asked why, she answered, "Mainly because you could get into a very long match and become very tired. Tennis isn't something you play quickly. It can go on for hours, and I think you take too big a risk."

However, one avid player said she never played as well as when she was pregnant: "Being pregnant heightens your awareness of your body. I had always had a problem with getting to the ball too soon. [Being pregnant] slowed me down a bit and everything fell into place. I could concentrate more and hit the ball better."

A lawyer from Minnesota said, "Initially I felt very comfortable, but I wasn't able to get around the court as my pregnancy progressed. I wasn't able to run very well toward the end, so I concentrated on my shots rather than scampering for the ball."

Notes.

- Don't feel you must exhibit an acute sense of competition, that you must play longer than you feel up to or go after balls that you shouldn't.

- Try not to overstretch when serving or smashing.

- Remember that when you are tired you begin to lose your reflexes.

- Don't play in excessive heat.

- Watch out for falls.

JOGGING AND RUNNING

Women are participating in jogging and running activities in increasing numbers, and for those runners who become pregnant there is no better advice than that offered by Nina Kuscsik, R.N. and fifty-mile marathon runner: "Each person must be aware of her own body. Do what you feel you want to, make adjustments based on how you feel, and modify your running program accordingly."

Try to keep up your regular program of running. In all likelihood, though, you'll have to modify it somewhat. One California banker who ran eight miles a week before she became pregnant cut back her activities 10 percent and was anticipating further cutbacks as she approached her eighth month.

In an article in *The Jogger,* the magazine of the National Jogging Association, Carol Dilfer, who runs the Prenatal/Postpartum Aerobics Fitness Program at the YMCA in Palo Alto, California, and who is the author of *Your Baby, Your Body,* offered in *The Jogger* some of the following suggestions for pregnant women runners, here condensed:

- Consult your physician.

- Plan a regular program of jogging, and do it at least three times a week.

- Begin each session with stretching exercises and a brief warm-up of major joint areas.

- Jog *gently*. If you cannot jog continually, alternate one minute of slow jogging with half a minute of walking. Maintain proper body mechanics when jogging—hold a good posture, land on the entire foot, hold hands loosely, wear proper running shoes.

- End each session with a cool-down period.

There are very few times when running or jogging cannot be helpful, but there are certain conditions in which you may be uncomfortable. These include:

Stress incontinence, in which you cannot control your bladder. Due to the pressure of the fetus on the stomach and kidneys, running may be inadvisable. "One thing about jogging," says a New York copywriter, "I'd go out and jog a little and inevitably I'd have to go. Even when my husband and I went hiking in the woods upstate one weekend I had to take Kleenex along because I just couldn't make it for two hours."

Jogger's nipples, which dozens of regular joggers complain of. This is a painful inflammation of the breasts, thought to be caused by a constant scraping of the chest against a shirt while running. To avoid "jogger's nipples," be sure to wear a bra or to coat the nipples with petroleum jelly when running. Wear an Ace bandage or double bra with wider straps to aid in supporting heavier breasts.

A rash in the crotch area, known as jock itch, which has afflicted men for years and is only now beginning to affect women. This may be particularly troublesome during pregnancy because of the moisture that tends to accumulate in the area. Try to keep the area as dry as possible and avoid any creams or ointments during the nine-month period.

A bad back. If you already have a bad back, pregnancy may aggravate it. Jogging may aggravate it even more. You may well want to discontinue this activity until after pregnancy. In any case, check with your doctor or ask

him to refer you to a sportsmedicine specialist or ortho-
pedic surgeon, who can discuss the pros and cons of
this activity—and your particular situation—with you
personally.

Running may help alleviate tired legs and varicose
veins, which many women experience during pregnancy.
Caused by pelvic congestion, these conditions may be
aided by running because it helps the blood to circulate
better.

Notes.

- Make sure you eat something prior to running, especially
  protein, to avoid faintness.

- Wear support stockings while running even though they may
  be a bit cumbersome.

- Try urinating immediately before you run in order to avoid
  stress incontinence during your exercise period.

SQUASH AND RACQUETBALL

Gretchen Spruance, national women's squash champion,
played squash singles until the fourth month of her pregnancy. "I probably would have continued," she says, "but
squash singles is a fast and furious game. Because of the
nature of the game you are stretching and twisting and
turning, and you have to be quick and move out of the
other person's way. I felt I was jarring myself and didn't
feel comfortable on the court, but I played up to that
point."

What did Spruance do to keep up her activity? Switched
to paddle tennis, squash doubles and tennis. "Squash
doubles is more like tennis," she said. "There is a larger
court, the stroke is more like tennis and it's a much
slower pace."

Spruance also said that she got out of breath faster,
so she watched the other person's racquet and relied
more on anticipation. "I got a little bit of a headstart,"
she said, "and it made me more aware of what the
other person was doing. I certainly was not as quick as
I had been."

Notes.

- Squash singles (as well as racquetball) is a very fast game, requiring continual concentration and movement, so you may want to consider squash doubles, paddle tennis or tennis after the first trimester.

- Check with your local club about playing while pregnant. Many limit play after the fourth month.

SWIMMING

"I swam and coached during my entire pregnancy," said Connie Roy, women's swimming coach at San Jose College and assistant coach, Santa Clara AAU Swim Club. "As a form of exercise I don't think there is anything better you can do."

Although swimming is one of the best forms of exercise for all 207 muscles of the body, it is the one sport that pregnant women worry most about. Questions about the risk of infection, water temperature and water entering the vaginal canal, especially during the last six weeks, are often heard.

Dr. Clayton Thomas, vice-president and medical affairs director of Tampax, Incorporated, and a member of the U.S. Olympic Sports Medicine Committee, addressed these issues: "It is virtually impossible for water to enter the vagina in ordinary swimming activity," he said. "Of all the body secretions, the vaginal secretions are the cleanest, so the likelihood of infection is small. If one is going to be infected, it is more likely that the infection will lodge in the ears or mouth, for instance. As far as water temperature, one should swim in whatever water temperature is most comfortable."

Dr. Thomas said, however, that such activities as water skiing and jumping feet first into the water are not recommended because of the forces produced when the body enters the water—and the possibility that water *could* be thrust upward into the vaginal canal in these circumstances.

In swimming, as in other sports, pacing is vital to the pregnant woman, says Connie Roy. "If one day she can do ten laps, that's fine; if the next day she can only do six laps, that's okay too. But it's good to try and do something every day."

Notes.

- While you are pregnant, pace yourself slower in swimming, especially if you are not used to the strain.

- Try swimming the breast stroke, which may be more comfortable than the freestyle.

- Avoid diving or jumping into the water feet first during the last few months because of the force with which the water might possibly enter the vagina.

BOWLING

As noted before, both Betty Morris and Cheryl Robinson, champion bowlers, agreed that their balance and timing was better during their pregnancies. Both felt that with the added weight, their approach to the line resulted in a slower delivery and more accurate release.

Notes.

- Try a heavier ball when you bowl to compensate for the added weight.

- Through the third trimester you may find it a bit difficult to bend over and may have to alter your approach somewhat.

- During breaks between games, drink milk instead of beer or soft drinks.

BICYCLE RIDING

If the weather is clear and dry, bike riding is one of the best forms of exercise for the pregnant woman. A racing bike may present some problems when you bend over, but if you have the sort of bike on which you can sit up, riding should not be uncomfortable at all.

Notes.

- Walk rather than ride up hills.

- Check the local terrain. If the ground is wet and slippery, it may be better to avoid cycling that day.

- Pull over when tired, and walk.

ICE SKATING

Depending on how expert a skater you are, this sport offers a range of possibilities. If you are a beginner, you may want to wear a heavy coat as a buffer against falls. Olympic champion Peggy Fleming skated throughout her pregnancy, and others have been known to accomplish sit spins as late as the eighth month.

Notes.

- Beware of falls.

- Because of the increased mammary development and concentration of abdominal weight, you may feel more off-balance while skating than during other sports.

- If you are skating outdoors, check the ice conditions first. Be sure you are wearing sharp skates.

FENCING

Because of the nature of the sport, fencing is one activity in which limited participation is recommended. Jan Romary, ten times national champion in foil for women and member of six Olympic teams, said, "When I found out I was pregnant, I stopped competing and took lessons— because in this particular sport you are poking a thirty-two-inch blade in someone's stomach."

In order to keep up her fencing activity, Romary fenced wearing a fencing master's plastron. This is a heavy canvas and leather vestlike protective garment, which cushions the blows. In addition, in her eighth and ninth months she avoided lunges.

Notes.

- Continue fencing through lessons rather than competition.

- Wear a protective covering over the abdomen, since this is part of the target area.

GYMNASTICS

Olympic gymnasts Cathy Rigby and Kim Chace (who was the highest scoring woman on the U.S. Gymnastics Team in 1976) said that they avoided work on the bars and high beams during their pregnancies. Both agreed that pregnant women who participate in gymnastics should keep away from stunts that are jarring to the body, such as back flips and aerial walkovers.

Recommended stunts and activities, depending on your physician's approval, include rolling tricks, handstands, cartwheels, and strength exercises, such as leg lifts and pull-ups. "As long as the movements are not jarring," Rigby says, "I see no reason why a woman couldn't continue with balletic movements as well."

Notes.

- Avoid any activity where you can easily fall, especially the bars and high beams.

- Remember that your reflexes may not be the same during pregnancy as prepregnancy.

HORSEBACK RIDING

More than any other, horseback riding is cited as the one activity that should be avoided during pregnancy. Why? Simply because in riding you depend to a large extent on the horse, and the risk of falls is great.

"Riding never bothered me," said Sally Ike, international equestrian champ, "but I did stop jumping at around seven months."

A New England dressage instructor and mother of six who rode and taught through each pregnancy (and who resumed riding five days after the birth of her sixth child) said, "I did dressage and low jumps, but my belly kept hitting the saddle on the high jumps, so I eliminated that. I was also a bit uncomfortable doing a sitting trot after my sixth month, so that went too.

"In every sport," she continued, "you can't be rash.

You can't ride for six hours. You have to be consistent and ride in moderation. If I overdid it, I had back problems and my legs hurt.

"I also did all the stable work, pitched hay and lugged buckets," she added.

When asked how her physician responded, she said, "He said to do what I was accustomed to doing. But he didn't know how much I was accustomed to doing, so I did everything."

Notes.

- If you have never ridden, do not begin now.

- It is probably better not to ride or train a new horse during this period.

- You may want to mount from a fence or stool rather than from the ground if your added weight causes you to be off-balance.

- Don't take risks you ordinarily wouldn't take.

GOLF

Golf involves twisting, with the emphasis on the torso. There is some disagreement among physicians about the extent to which it should be played, especially in the latter months of pregnancy. Nevertheless, many women, both pros and amateurs, have played golf during their pregnancies, competitively and socially.

Susie Maxwell Berning, winner of the U.S. Women's Open in 1968, 1972 and 1973, played through the better part of her two pregnancies. "After the fifth month I had to flatten my swing," she said, "in order to compensate for my belly. After that I couldn't play competitively, but I played for fun and had a great time."

Berning described her short game, or the shots involving chipping and putting, as "jerky," but she still played twice a week during most of the nine-month period, stopping only when the heat became excessive.

"I kept waiting for things to happen and nothing did, so I just kept playing," said a woman golfer from Atlanta

who won her club championship when she was eight
months pregnant. "I had to succumb to using a cart, but
that was because of the added weight."

Many women have cited the walking involved in playing
the game as excellent exercise. As the pregnancy moves
toward the third trimester, the pregnant golfer may experience difficulty putting, and may have to limit her swing.
Once again, with common sense she may be able to play
virtually up to the point of delivery.

Notes.

- Avoid playing in excessive heat.
- Use a golf cart when walking or carrying clubs makes you
  uncomfortable.
- Avoid full swings.
- Leave your wooden clubs home.

SKIING

In skiing, the pregnant woman should beware of high-
speed falls (and a possible broken limb). "In alpine skiing
especially," says Herman Goellner, head coach of the
U.S. Women's Alpine Ski Team, "if the person is challenge oriented, the potential for falls exists."

Goellner suggests that pregnant women who ski should
do so one step below their normal level in intermediate
terrain and under good snow conditions. He also suggests
that because skiing is generally considered to be a sprint
sport, the pregnant skier should consider switching to
cross-country skiing for the duration of the pregnancy, as
the latter is more of an aerobic sport.

One woman who normally skis at the intermediate
level said she felt lightheaded during one downhill run.
She laid down in the snow until she regained her compo-
sure, skied to the bottom and called it a day. "The air felt
terrific," she said, "but after that I definitely skied more
passively."

Notes.

- Take note of snow conditions. If the snow is filled with
  moguls and ice it is probably better to stay away.

- Be aware of changes in gravity—your balance may shift backward.

- Avoid excessive exertion by skiing one level below your normal ability.

There are other sports in which women have participated during their pregnancies, but in fewer numbers than those mentioned above. Pregnant women have played softball ("I had the baby on Friday and returned to play the following Friday"), scuba dived and even ridden steers in a rodeo competition.

If you are in doubt, ask your physician or medical support team and use your common sense. If your physician is negative or unknowledgeable about participation in a particular sport, call the local college or high school and ask for one of the women's athletic trainers or physicians. Request the name of a medical person who knows about your particular sport, and have your own physician consult with the expert about the effect your physical activity might have on your pregnancy. If you are in good health and are experiencing a normal pregnancy, you have a right to know why physical activity may not be recommended for you.

Outmoded attitudes toward physical activity during pregnancy are beginning to change, but it is still early in the game. Sportsmedicine specialists can give advice, women pros can set examples, and trainers and coaches can help the pregnant woman learn how her body responds. The real effort, however, will come from women themselves. Dr. Hale summed it up when he said, "In the future, women are not going to accept no's from physicians in areas where there is not only interest, but activity as well."

4

TRAVEL

Healthy pregnant women can

- Fly in airplanes
- Cruise on wonderful ships
- Tour foreign lands
- Run meetings, see clients, close deals, and do business thousands of miles from home

Whether or not they *do* depends on necessity, desire and attitude—their own and the world's.

"Few, if any, pregnant women in their right minds travel. You should have seen the faces—I won't even repeat the comments when I raised the question in our office," exclaimed the advertising manager of a major cruise line when questioned. "If you want to write about something, why don't you ask me what really happens on a singles' cruise. Now, there's a story!"

He's wrong—wrong even about his own industry.

Two women executives for rival cruise lines—both holding jobs similar to his—traveled by air and sea during their recent pregnancies. One of these women did marketing surveys in Atlanta, Los Angeles, Boston and Houston while pregnant, and cruised to Bermuda in her third month. She said, "I found that I did even better at sea. I didn't stand out. If I had morning sickness, other people

102

were seasick. If I ordered special foods, the dining-room staff is used to catering to different diets. The wine steward automatically brought me two Cokes every time I sat down at the table, because I had ordered them the first night out to settle my stomach. My husband and some people we both knew were on the ship. While they were nervous about me, I was just fine. I did the work that I had to do—we were starting a new route and I had to know all about it to help sell it. After work I was free to nap, have a late dinner and dance until all hours. Even when we hit one night of very rough seas and I thought, 'Why did I do this to myself?' I knew the answer. It would pass, and being on a ship was a lot better than being stuck in an office."

You don't have to be a travel professional to leave home during pregnancy. One Boston woman works for an educational testing service and travels 40 percent of her time. Pregnancy made no difference. She commuted between Boston and Washington every other week of her pregnancy and ran a seminar in Denver. A pregnant Californian visited her husband's family in Germany. A New York graduate student who rarely has money for travel and who dislikes flying had a week with her husband in St. Lucia during her fourth month. She swam and walked and reveled on that lushly green island with pleasure and without problems. She also made a discovery en route. She said, "Because of my pregnancy, I didn't want to use Dramamine, so I went on the plane expecting to be horribly sick. Instead, I never felt better. Thanks to my baby, I learned that I'll never have to depend on airsickness drugs again."

Women who have traveled while pregnant start out feeling that they are doing something special, adventurous and unusual. To a certain extent they are.

"You're crazy, go home" was the comment one pregnant tourist heard often from other Americans that she met while in Greece; the Greeks that she met just smiled and wished her luck. When the wife of a leading U.S. space scientist went to Russia during her first pregnancy, people in Red Square stopped to stare. She thought that the attraction was her obvious belly. "I was wrong," she recalled with a laugh. "They were staring at my raincoat. It was bright yellow, made of shiny plastic. In all of Russia, raincoats only come in black, tan or brown. They had seen plenty of pregnant women, but they hadn't seen anything like my raincoat before!"

Pregnant travelers need a sense of humor and spunk, because they often must cross a frontier of misinformation and a barrier of regulations as tangled as barbed wire.

MEDICAL FACTS ABOUT TRAVEL

With an understanding of what to expect and with careful planning and medical approval, healthy pregnant women can and do travel well. There are some pregnant women who should absolutely not travel. There are some times during pregnancy when it is better to travel than at other times. Some modes of travel are preferable to others.

Generally, however, the situation is as Dr. Warren Pearse, executive director of the American College of Obstetricians and Gynecologists, describes it: "There is not much that you can do to harm either the mother or baby through traveling. The hazards of travel during pregnancy are largely overrated." Occasionally, an obstetrician will joke: "Sure, you can go, but you have to take your obstetrician along for a vacation."

The unborn baby exists within the best protective packaging on earth. This was made very clear during World War II in studies comparing the rates of abortion, premature labor and other obstetric complications among pregnant women who traveled with their husbands in military service to those of pregnant military wives who stayed put. There was no significant difference in their childbearing experiences.

In the last five years, some obstetricians have noted an increase in the number of pregnant patients asking clearance to travel. It's no real surprise. More and more women have to travel for business. When it comes to pleasure trips and vacations, the travel industry wisely aims much of its sales pitch directly at women, because women are prime decision makers about if, when and where a couple or family will go. The fact that many women love to travel is clear.

A Manhattan legal secretary, who brown-bags lunch every day to save money for the two yearly trips abroad that she and her husband take, explained, "One of the women lawyers in my firm went to the Orient when she was pregnant, and the thought frightened me so much that I was sure that something would happen to the baby. She came back in great shape and so happy that I decided that the fear of traveling pregnant wasn't as bad as my fear of being stuck home for nine months!"

A woman who is worried or afraid to travel during pregnancy—a woman who would blame herself forever if an obstetrical crisis that might well have occurred at home happened during a trip—is a prime candidate for staying close to home. Women who travel well and successfully during pregnancy often have a trait in common: confidence in the rightness and safety of what they are doing. But a woman who isn't altogether happy about the idea of traveling during pregnancy shouldn't force herself. Travel means added excitement, new experiences, different environment and, often, questionable food. If you are healthy and want to travel, these stress factors are acceptable, and the pleasure of travel can add to the enjoyment of your pregnancy. If you really don't want to travel, you are just adding unnecessary strain.

Travel during pregnancy isn't for every woman for reasons other than fear. Complicating medical conditions, such as diabetes or heart disease, or any high-risk obstetrical factor, such as a history of miscarriage or the possibility of twins, are valid reasons behind a medical order to stay home.

If you want to travel, it is important to have a complete discussion with your physician or health team as soon in pregnancy as possible, because early hints of such problems as hypertension can be taken into account. The strategy of medical care abroad can be set, and the question of immunization can be discussed. It also helps the pregnant traveler's peace of mind to have a checkup just before leaving and immediately upon returning home.

The very best time to travel during pregnancy is the second trimester, when the statistical risk of miscarriage or premature labor is the lowest and when many women feel fine. Travel very late in pregnancy is actively discouraged, and the travel industry does its best to refuse soon-to-be mothers. The notion is dramatic, but few babies today are born on shipboard or above the clouds.

THE QUESTION OF FLYING DURING PREGNANCY

More than any other form of travel, flying raises questions for pregnant women. Most everyone worries that being thousands of feet above the earth and zooming through clouds will prompt a miscarriage, start labor or harm an unborn child in some way.

For answers, we have to turn to the experiences of flight attendants and the observations of medical scientists, including aerospace physicians. We are going to review the medical assessments of the pregnant woman flier to underline findings relevant to you, the pregnant passenger.

The question is, What can harm you or your baby if you fly? The answer is, The same things that can harm any other passenger, that is, a hijacking, an emergency landing or an equipment problem. These are remote risks any air traveler must assume but will probably not experience.

What, then, is special about flying that might harm your baby? In flying, as in mountain climbing, a condition can occur called hypoxia, or oxygen deprivation. In theory, hypoxia is dangerous to a pregnant woman because a good oxygen supply is vital to her baby. In actuality, the danger doesn't exist because today's commercial aircraft have pressurized cabins. If there is a problem and cabin pressure drops, oxygen masks descend to ensure adequate oxygen. Dr. R. Graeme Cameron, a Swiss physician who has studied the effects of work on flight attendants in the first trimester, has written, "There is no evidence that either flying per se or the hypoxia induced at cabin altitude of five thousand to seven thousand feet has any deleterious effect on mother, embryo or fetus."

As for other supposed hazards of flying, Dr. Paul

Scholten of the University of California Medical School in San Francisco wrote in *Aviation Space and Environmental Medicine* that "Flying offers no great abortion hazard save that of trauma and trauma is an unusual cause of abortion. A certain number of pregnant women will begin or finish an abortion while flying, and being human, will blame flying as the cause. Almost without exception, flying will have nothing to do with abortion, except as the scene of the drama." Dr. Scholten, who also discussed the effects of irregular rest and sleep patterns of pregnant flight attendants, noted that "there is no known direct action from these irregularities on the developing fetus."

If you still have qualms about the safety of flying, you may be reassured to know that some U.S. airlines have changed their rulings to permit flight attendants to work during the first six months of pregnancy. Prior to this change, flight attendants were forced to go on an unpaid leave as soon as pregnancy was discovered. As a result, women who wanted or needed work were forced to fly as long as they could, covering the evidence of pregnancy with loose clothing. We interviewed flight attendants who worked with the knowledge of management, and several who flew with hidden passengers. Said one who hid her pregnancy and worked aloft: "My own doctor felt that it was quite safe and much healthier for me to keep working, because I was getting all the exercise and activity that I am used to."

As a pregnant passenger, all of the above facts should dispel any doubts that you may have. As a passenger, however, you should know that there are a variety of airline regulations that apply to you during pregnancy. These will be fully discussed on pages 113–14.

WHY TRAVEL?

Travel during pregnancy has special benefits.

If it is a pleasure trip, it can be what Dr. Charles Bauer, clinical associate professor of pediatrics at the Cornell–New York Medical Center and an author of a book aimed at new mothers, calls "the last free time. If they travel after that, the parents will always worry about the child left at home." If you are contemplating travel in a repeat pregnancy, Dr. Bauer notes that this is best done before a child is six months old or much later, when children can understand what is happening and that their parents will return—a crucial point.

If it is a trip for a pregnant woman with several other children, it can be a blessed relief. When a pregnant travel agent in the Midwest went to her obstetrician for a checkup and an okay to keep flying, he said, "I wish my other pregnant women, the ones with four other kids to take care of, had your job and a chance to get away."

If it is business travel, the willingness and ability to do what one has to during pregnancy means job protection and is proof of serious intent to continue a career. For example, the director of a giant advertising agency's international offices worked hard and long in New York headquarters to prepare a week-long meeting for key people from European offices to be held in Brussels. The fact that the meeting coincided with the start of her eighth month didn't concern her, although top brass felt that somehow it was improper for a naturally slim woman carrying an enormous belly to travel and run an important meeting. Her obstetrician gave her three rules: "One, when you are on the plane, make sure that you get up and walk around once an hour. Two, never skip a meal, and if you can't have a proper meal, eat lightly several times a day. Three, if you go into labor, the people who arranged the meeting for you can get you competent help. If you have a question at any time, for God's sake, pick up the phone and call me."

Allowing herself only the luxury of having her husband travel with her (he was delighted to go), but easing her professional conscience by adding on three days of work in Paris after the meeting, she flew to Belgium. None of her overseas colleagues knew that she was pregnant, and when she waddled in, "either they were too embarrassed or too indifferent to say anything. Privately, some of the men said that they thought I was terrific." The meetings ran from nine in the morning to six at night. She gave presentations sitting down, and took a nap in the early evenings. Traveling while pregnant proved to herself and to her colleagues the seriousness of her intention to retain her career. She also experienced some of the unexpected dividends when the owner of a restaurant, with a courtly nod to her belly, offered a gift of wine and a toast "for the baby." And back in the States she had a healthy son, full term.

A PREGNANT WOMAN'S BAEDECKER: WHERE TO GO, HOW TO GO

If you have a choice, you should have your travel plans custom-tailored to your desires, with safety factors in line with past travel experience. Pregnancy is not the time for a first cruise or for a beginning traveler to try to manage a visit to a country where it is rare to find someone who speaks English or where lodgings are uncomfortable.

If you have never left the United States, a pregnancy trip might be most enjoyable in Great Britain, where there is no language hurdle, where medical facilities are excellent, and where it is highly unlikely that you will consume food and drink carrying those evil things that cause traveler's diarrhea. If you are an experienced traveler and you opt for exotic travel, it is still important to plan each day's itinerary to include proper rest. The excitement of fabulous sights or the desire to keep up can fire you into doing more than is comfortable. Pregnant women have to guard against becoming overtired wherever they go.

YOUR FOOD NEEDS ABROAD

Unless nations are known to be absolutely strict about hygiene standards, it is smart to drink bottled water, avoid ice cubes and use tap water for tooth-brushing only after running it hot for a while. Stored water on trains, buses or airplanes should be avoided. The rest of the world may be insulted or amused at the American preoccupation with sanitation, but safe food and drink are essential for you because you are trying to avoid the use of medication. The body needs plenty of fluid, especially during travel, but the fluid should be free of potential problems. This means boiled tea or coffee and bottled water or soft drinks, provided that they are purchased with an unopened seal or cap.

Since pasteurized milk may not be available (and some milk is improperly pasteurized despite the label), it is better to avoid milk and milk products, such as yogurt or ice cream. Hard cheese is a safe form of milk protein and nutrients. Two other options for milk: (1) Pack a supply of powdered dry skim milk, which can be used in coffee or tea or can be reconstituted with bottled water; or (2) buy canned evaporated or condensed milk abroad and add boiled or bottled water.

It is advisable to avoid all fresh fruits except those that can be peeled, and to eat only cooked vegetables. Meats should be well cooked. Raw shellfish has a hepatitis potential. When you travel, the world is your oyster, so leave the real oyster alone.

Given the above precautions, you might think that pregnant women travel on empty stomachs, which is far from true. In fact, one of the more common admonitions of obstetricians before a patient leaves is, "Don't gain too much weight."

PACKING YOUR SUITCASE

Whether a fledgling or experienced traveler, in pregnancy you should journey prepared. Here's what one woman packed for a six-week trip through Europe: "Dry milk packets lined my suitcase; I had extra supplies of my vitamins and iron, simple medications for colds and diarrhea (my doctor recommended paregoric rather than Lomotil) that I could use safely if needed; a small inflatable pillow for the small of my back, which was a great help on buses and trains; loose, comfortable clothing that wouldn't make me look silly in another culture (no binding pantsuits) and would still fit six weeks later; and the Guttmacher book on pregnancy to use as a reference, so that I could distinguish between a possible warning signal and a normal event."

Pregnant travelers should carry phrase books and small foreign-language dictionaries (which often are more useful). The most important word to know in another language is "toilet." The most useful phrases are "I am in my —— month"; "This is my —— child"; "I feel very well, thank you."

FINDING HELP FAR FROM HOME

Here again, it is essential to travel prepared, with a firm idea of who to contact and where to go if you need medical attention or even if you just want to speak with a physician. This means preparation before leaving home. For domestic trips, obstetricians have source books listing colleagues all over the country, and should be able to supply names. Thanks to their own travel experiences and to their training, during which they may have met foreign medical students, many obstetricians have friends abroad. The International Association for Medical Assistance to Travelers (Suite 5620, Empire State Building, 350 Fifth Avenue, New York, New York 10001) will supply (for a donation) an international directory of physicians abroad who have been trained in English-speaking countries.

Abroad, the major hotel chains, such as Hilton, can refer you to an English-speaking doctor even if you are not a hotel guest. So can the ubiquitous American Express offices. It is always useful to have a letter from your obstetrician, detailing due date, blood type and any particular health conditions.

IMMUNIZATIONS

The U.S. Public Health Service maintains the renowned Center for Disease Control (Atlanta, Georgia 30333), which is a traveler's best friend. The Center keeps local health departments informed of disease outbreaks around the world in weekly bulletins. If, for example, the Caribbean island you have selected for a vacation is reporting polio, the Center will know about it. If you have a question about whether you should be immunized during your pregnancy, either you or your obstetrician can check with the Center.

In 1973 ACOG issued a technical bulletin discussing immunization during pregnancy. Unfortunately, there is incomplete information about the effects of vaccines and some diseases on pregnant women. If there is a choice of where to travel and if there is a question about the safety of vaccine, you may be wiser to change your destination than to be vaccinated. This is especially true when the vaccine contains a live virus. Pregnant women are advised against travel in areas where plague, yellow fever or smallpox is endemic. Polio vaccine is indicated only for susceptible women traveling in areas where it is endemic. Flu vaccine should be used at the discretion of your physician. If an area is reporting measles, German measles or mumps, you should avoid travel there. Protective vaccines themselves can injure the fetus.

IF YOU GO BY AIR

The good news about traveling by air while pregnant is that some pregnant passengers get "bumped" into first class if there's room and if the flight personnel are kind. Also, obstetricians recommend air travel over long-distance car trips. With advance planning, a pregnant passenger can request bulkhead seats on the aircraft, which generally are more roomy. You can also preorder the most suitable meals.

The bad, but not so bad, news about flight during pregnancy is that airlines have a maze of rules regarding the transport of pregnant women, and can create an unpleasant hassle at the gate or even refuse to board you. Some airlines will board a woman near term only when she has special medical clearance, and a woman in labor only if there is reason to transport her to better medical facilities and no air ambulance is available. Although babies have been safely born high in the sky (one infant thereby earning a free lifetime ticket on its natal airline), flight personnel have usually had only the bare minimum training in emergency childbirth.

It makes life infinitely easier to have an obstetrician's note stating due date and fitness to travel. The note is particularly useful if you are "carrying big" and airline employees may think you are ready to give birth at the ticket counter. A pregnant woman may take ten flights during her pregnancy and may be bothered or questioned or challenged on only one small connecting flight; still, it's a good idea to be prepared. Some airlines require a pregnant woman to sign a legal release form.

Whenever one flies while pregnant it is essential for you or your travel agent to double-check regulations because they can change almost as quickly as fares! Here is a sampling of domestic and international airline rules in alphabetical order:

American Airlines	Can board any time until seven days before due date.
British Airways	On overseas flights from United States, pregnant passenger must have physician's note if more than four months pregnant.
Air France	After eighth month, physician's note is necessary.
Delta	No proof of stage of pregnancy is formally required; however, they will not allow a passenger to fly if she looks "unhealthy."
Eastern	Can board through eighth month, but requires physician's letter in ninth month to fly up to two weeks before due date; may refuse passenger if she looks close to delivery.
Japan Airlines	No restrictions through eighth month. In ninth month must have JAL form letter signed by physician seventy-two hours before departure. Due date and special medical conditions must be included.
KLM–Royal Dutch	After thirty-fourth week, physician's name and telephone number is required to contact for approval.

Lufthansa (German)	Until twenty-eighth week, physician's note is required that states delivery is not anticipated in the next four weeks. Will not accept pregnant passengers from eighth month on.
National	Not allowed to board in ninth month.
Northwest Orient	Eighth and ninth months, physician's letter is necessary.
Ozark	Pregnant passenger is allowed to buy ticket; however, at any time pilot has the right to refuse her to fly.
Pan American	After thirty-fifth week, physician's letter is necessary.
Qantas (Australian)	No restriction up to thirty-five weeks; thereafter, they require letter from passenger's physician or certificate from airline physician stating that passenger is able to fly.
SAS (Scandinavian)	Accepts pregnant passengers through eighth month; refused in ninth month.
Transworld	Will not accept a pregnant passenger after the start of eighth month without a physician's note. (Infants must be seven days old before they can be taken on a flight.)
United	In the eighth month of pregnancy, passenger must have obstetrician's certification dated within seventy-two hours of flight departure stating that an examination has been made and the woman is fit to travel from point of departure to destination. Expected delivery date must be included.

Most airlines will assign better seats to pregnant passengers if requested in advance. Some women may wish to request seats near bathrooms. If requested, preferably in advance, most airlines will provide luggage assistance or wheelchairs for covering the endless corridors that are part of the modern airport scene. Some airlines are less gracious to pregnant women than others.

Once on an airplane, you have a major task: You must be sure to walk during the flight. When seated, keep your feet elevated. Pregnancy slows blood circulation and sitting too long in one position can promote the formation of harmful blood clots. As for seat belts, they should be worn fairly loose, fastened under the womb, over your lap. Since feet and ankles may swell on a flight, it's not a good idea to take your shoes off because they may not fit on landing. On the ground, swollen ankles will subside if legs are rested up on a chair.

For extra comfort and ease on a flight, eye shades and ear plugs can be an aid to sleep. As for jet lag, pregnant flight attendants and airline medical directors recommend sleeping for three or four hours on landing and then forcing yourself to get up and function in a new time zone. Even though there is a temptation to eat, drink and be merry aboard a flight, it is better to eat lightly and drink little to help the body adjust to a new environment and time zone.

What if obstetrical problems arise en route? While airlines do their utmost to avoid carrying a woman with a near-term baby, and a pregnant woman may fantasize about having the world's greatest obstetrician no more than a seat away, the responsibility falls to flight attendants. Some are trained to administer first aid in case of miscarriage; some have seen movies or slides of delivery; some have no training in emergency childbirth; some have training; others have been taught that if labor starts they are to (1) page the airplane for medical personnel aboard, and (2) discuss with the captain the possibility of emergency landing near medical facilities. Most major airports have medical facilities with nurses on duty and physicians on call.

If You Go By Sea

Sea travel—transport or cruising—offers the pregnant traveler several attractive features: It is a relaxing way to travel; activity can be scheduled at one's own pace; there are fine ship-to-shore communications; food selection is possible; and above all else, there is access to medical care.

On the downside, it is important to realize that accidental injury can occur on rough seas; medical facilities can vary greatly; and sea travel is not a good idea if a pregnant woman hasn't sailed before. Your decision about whether or not you want to travel by sea depends in part on your worries about seasickness. In recent years, the problems of seasickness for all passengers has lessened because of the use of modern ship stabilizers, which eliminate side-to-side roll. There is, however, the motion of going up and over waves, which can also create seasickness, particularly in bad seas. Can you deal with this problem while you are pregnant? According to Dr. P. O. Oliver, group medical director of the Cunard Lines, "Pregnancy does tend to increase the probability and intensity of seasickness." This is a general statement, and in making up your mind about sea travel you should know that we interviewed many women who cruised during pregnancy successfully without seasickness problems; and of those who did experience seasickness many said it was controllable. If you have a choice, you can cruise in waters known for calmness at a particular time of the year. By selecting a cabin in the middle of the ship, regardless of deck, you can minimize motion problems.

Women who have cruised during pregnancy report that saltines and other forms of carbohydrates are useful seasickness antidotes, but the best medicine of all is deep breathing on the open deck. Heavy meals and drinking can lead to discomfort.

Some obstetricians will prescribe motion-sickness medicine and ship doctors may offer medication in tablet or injectable form. In any case, ask if there are contraindications or identifiable risks for pregnant women. The no-drugs-during-pregnancy rule is the best to follow. (See the discussion of the anti-nausea drug, Bendectin, in Chapter Five.)

Whereas such a ship as the *Queen Elizabeth II* carries a hospital capable of serving some three thousand passengers and crew, complete with an incubator and doctors and nurses who have midwifery training, staff and facilities vary greatly from ship to ship. Passenger ships are required to have a physician aboard, but, depending on the country of origin, the physician may not speak English although other staff should be available for translation. Ships are prepared to give emergency first aid and to leave passengers at hospitals in ports en route rather than to attempt elective surgery or serious treatment at sea. Cargo ships with less than a given number of passengers may not have the medical facilities of cruise ships.

Rules governing pregnant sea travelers vary. One line may require that pregnant passengers register with the ship's doctor. Fairly typical are lines such as Holland American or Home Lines, which require obstetrician clearance to accept a pregnant woman from the sixth month on. The Home Lines requests a consultation between ship-and-shore physicians as well.

If You Go By Car or Bus

Whether as commuters, pleasure travelers or car-pool mothers, pregnant women are on the road. This raises the seat-belt question. For example, a real-estate broker spent most of her second pregnancy driving customers to houses and properties. A pregnant law student drove thirty-five miles each way to law school and then added another ten miles each day commuting to a part-time job as a law clerk. The realtor couldn't be bothered with seat belts, the law student always wore one. Who was right?

In a pamphlet bluntly entitled *Safety Belts for People Who Enjoy Living*, the Automobile Association of America states "Safety belts make good sense for the pregnant passenger . . . safety belts may put pressure on the mother and her unborn child in a crash. But that pressure is much less harmful than being slammed against the inside of the car if she doesn't wear belts. In older cars with separate lap and shoulder belts, both should be worn, with the lap belt adjusted snugly and low across the abdomen."

In a study of auto accidents by the Department of Obstetrics and Gynecology at the Royal Women's Hospital in Melbourne, Australia, in those cases where both the

mother and unborn baby died the woman was not wearing a seat belt. In some instances, a waist seat belt may
protect the mother from serious head or chest injuries,
but may also contribute to uterine injury in the case of an
accident. Therefore, if possible use the shoulder-strap
variety.

Since car breakdowns may be an added bother during
pregnancy, these nine months are a good time to be sure
that everything automotive is in tune all the time, and to
avoid side roads not in good repair. Use main roads in
foreign countries, and rent a larger car rather than the
smallest available. Except in late pregnancy when labor
is imminent, car travel—even long distance—is possible.
However, most physicians advise pregnant women to break
up car trips at least every two hours for the same reason
women are advised to walk during long airplane flights. A
back pillow can also be a comfort on a long trip.

As for long-distance bus rides, the Greyhound Bus
Lines reports no rules, regulations or problems with trans-
porting pregnant passengers. Although bus drivers have
no training in childbirth, they have been known to help
deliver babies, and, of course, they can drive a woman to
proper help. Pregnant women who may have questions
about long hours on a tour bus may gain some insight
from a travel agent who had to test a tour of Ireland as
part of her job in her fourth month. She said, "The bus
was deluxe, the roads were fine, it was so much better
than the terrible jostling I imagined. And it certainly beat
commuting to work back home, because at least on the
tour bus I got a seat!"

When it comes to accepting pregnant tourists, large
operators, such as American Express or Thomas Cook,
note that they are bound by airline rules and regulations.
Also, as the American Express brochures make very clear,
some tours involve a lot of walking, have busy schedules
and will not be enjoyed by those unable to keep up. Tour
leaders are usually not able to give first aid, but often
have been trained in how to get medical help quickly in
foreign lands.

Tour operators questioned note that pregnant tourists
are uncommon. Somehow, the world is able to nod at a

pregnant business traveler, army wife or cruise passenger sitting in a deck chair, but who imagines a sightseeing pregnant tourist? Nonetheless, pregnant women *can* be very successful tourists. In her sixth month, a Florida bank officer toured Spain. She said, "There were times when my husband had to help push me up on the bus, but within reason I saw it all: the incredible beauty of Granada, bullfights in Madrid, the hills of Toledo. It was extraordinary to explore new places while I was pregnant and to know that our love of travel didn't have to be sacrificed just because we were expecting a baby. Some-day we'll take our child to Spain too!" Contrary to stay-at-home tradition, pregnant women are proving that travel, adventure and the great fun of a change of scene can easily be part of the New Pregnancy.

Bon voyage.

5

ACHIEVING A HEALTHY PREGNANCY

Enough is known about the impact of our habits of food, drink and drugs on the fetus that for many women pregnancy means changing some trustworthy or convenient ways of living. If this is your first pregnancy, you may hear some no's that you never expected; if this is a repeat pregnancy, you may need some new information, because in the world of obstetrics there is always change and controversy. For example, supplemental vitamins are widely prescribed by obstetricians, but may not be needed. Or where once our mothers were advised not to gain too much weight, today's obstetrician advises you to gain at least twenty-four to twenty-six pounds. We are urged to eat well—that our babies will literally be what we consume—and not to diet.

You will have to make some changes in such habits as smoking, taking pills and going on crash diets. But this is a chance for you to exert control over what happens to you and your baby. You can actually *do* something that can make a vast difference, and you may develop a good health habit or two as a bonus.

However, you may find that changing familiar patterns may bring unwelcome stress and tension. Therefore, we'll offer suggestions to help you make these changes in a comfortable way.

We're going to review some recent findings and facts

important to you, and suggest ways to integrate needed change into the rhythm of your life: how, for example, to adapt nutritional requirements to business lunches or stops at the local junk-food drive-in with your other kids; what to do about drugs and alcohol; and how to cope with the environment.

FOOD—THE NUTRITIONAL ASPECTS OF PREGNANCY

You are pregnant at a time of national mania about nutrition, when health food stores are flourishing, when women and men are popping megavitamins, and when some pregnant women are strongly committed to vegetarianism. You are also pregnant at a time when the obstetrical world has changed its mind about diet, weight gain and salt restriction.

Many women hate to gain weight, and associate pregnancy with all of the unhappy problems of being fat. Other women find themselves, after pregnancy, with an obesity problem that can linger unconquered for years. This situation doesn't call for dieting during pregnancy. It does mean knowing some of the basics of nutrition in pregnancy—why you need what, and how much—and some of the psychology of eating during pregnancy.

Good nutrition is one of the most important gifts that you can give yourself and your baby. If you don't give it, your baby will make every effort to take what it needs from what you eat or from your body. It's no surprise to find in a medical journal an ad for supplemental iron pills that shows a large color photograph of a fetus in the womb with a headline that shouts in large type: THIEF!

Pregnancy is a process of continuous dynamic growth—and growth demands energy. Two microscopic cells merge, and nine months later a baby kicks and cries with independent life. That kind of production requires about 300 calories a day above the intake normal for your age, height, body build and general level of activity, and varies according to where you are in pregnancy. It demands a balance of nutrients and supplements when needed. Your physician may suggest modifications based on your medical condition and prepregnancy weight; however, the best information available today says that a marked caloric restriction at this time in your life may harm you and your baby.

Poor maternal nutrition is strongly associated with low-birth-weight babies. This became clear during World War II. In the winter of 1944–45 food was scarce, and near-starvation was suffered by pregnant women in the Netherlands, who gave birth to lower birth-weight babies. Good maternal nutrition, on the other hand, is strongly associated with a satisfactory pregnancy outcome. By way of contrast to the sad situation in the Netherlands, in Great Britain it was possible to amend the food-rationing policy to give special attention to pregnant women. Despite the hazardous conditions of wartime Britain, the nation's stillbirth rate dropped because pregnant women were given the nutrition they required. What this means to you is that your proper, steady weight gain is an index of the health of your pregnancy.

Today it is becoming increasingly apparent that a woman's nutritional history from childhood is important to her nutritional status during pregnancy. Obviously, there is great concern about poor women and teen-agers who begin pregnancy in deprived nutritional states. Less obvious is the fact that many middle- and upper-class women can also be poorly nourished, through choice (fad dieting) or lack of information. As research for this book has shown, the medical advice given to pregnant women about nutrition can vary from almost zero to informed help. "When I asked my doctor about nutrition," one pregnant woman said, "he just looked at me—I was well dressed and I wear good jewelry—and he said, 'Just go ahead with what you are doing. You don't look like a junk-food eater to me.' And that was that."

Assess Your Nutritional Status

To learn how you stack up nutritionally during pregnancy means more than looking at a scale. As we all know, the term "empty calories" doesn't refer to air; it means potato chips and other foods that efficiently add weight to your body and do nothing for your baby. Unless your health team is willing to go over your nutritional status with you, you should do it yourself. With proper nutrition you will be better able to cope with the stress of pregnancy, you may avoid some complications and you may deal more successfully with labor and delivery. Your baby will more likely be born at term and in good health, and will do well in infancy. Proper nutrition means that you will show a slow, steady pattern of weight gain, and that you will have a good balance of essential nutrients with supplementation when necessary.

To assess your status, keep a diary of everything that you are currently eating for several days or a week. Then make some comparisons between what you are consuming and what is required, as listed in the following maternity nutrition chart, which was prepared by the March of Dimes. The chart is useful because it explains the importance of various nutrients in pregnancy and their most common or best sources (for the special nutritional requirements for adolescent pregnancy, check your local March of Dimes chapter).

Maternity Nutrition Plan

THE FOODS YOU AND YOUR BABY NEED	HOW MUCH EACH DAY?	WHY?
Milk . . . whole evaporated, skim, dry or buttermilk; hard, semi-soft, and cottage cheeses; yogurt. Soybean milk and soybean curd (tofu) may be substituted if Vitamin B-12, in which they are deficient, is taken in another form.	4 servings each day; 5 servings for breast feeding. Part can be in cream soups, cocoa, custard, or puddings.	Milk helps build strong bones and teeth. It helps nerves and muscles react normally, aids clotting of blood, and helps make the body run at peak efficiency. Milk contains many vitamins, protein, and minerals, such as calcium, zinc, magnesium, and phosphorus.

Maternity Nutrition Plan

THE FOODS YOU AND YOUR BABY NEED	HOW MUCH EACH DAY?	WHY?
Protein Foods . . . Animal: meat, poultry, liver, fish, eggs, milk. Vegetable: beans, peas, nuts, soybean curd (tofu), peanut butter.	4 servings each day; same for breast feeding. A serving is 2 to 3 ounces of cooked lean solid meat, poultry, or fish. Protein alternates: ¾ cup cooked dry beans, peas, or lentils; ¼ cup peanut butter; or 1 ounce of nuts.	Protein is the basic building material for you and your baby. It builds and repairs all tissues and helps make hemoglobin for blood and forms antibodies to fight infection. Protein supplies energy and helps your fetus develop and grow strong.
Leafy Green Vegetables . . . spinach, kale, dark leafy lettuces, broccoli, chard, collard and other greens, Brussels sprouts, asparagus, bok choy, cabbage, watercress, etc.	2 servings each day; same for breast feeding. A serving is 1 cup raw or ¾ cup cooked.	Needed to develop your baby's skeleton and his eyes, skin, hair, teeth, gums, and glands. Helps keep your skin and hair healthy. Necessary for good vision.
Vitamin C-Rich Fruits and Vegetables . . . oranges, grapefruit, mango, papaya, strawberries, tangerine, pineapple, tomato, green, red or chili peppers, cabbage, bok choy, Brussels sprouts, broccoli, cauliflower.	1 serving each day; same for breast feeding. Use fresh, frozen, or canned. Since Vitamin C cannot be stored in the body, be sure to have a fruit, vegetable, or juice from this group daily.	Vitamin C is needed to form healthy bones, teeth, and gums. It helps build strong body cells and blood vessels; also helps in healing wounds.
Other Fruits and Vegetables . . . carrots, potatoes, sweet potatoes, yams, squash, hominy, pea pods, mushrooms,	1 serving each day; same for breast feeding. Have a salad and/or raw fruit nibbles every day. For example, if	Yellow fruits and vegetables have Vitamin A, essential for both mother and fetus. This group also

Maternity Nutrition Plan

THE FOODS YOU AND YOUR BABY NEED	HOW MUCH EACH DAY?	WHY?
bean sprouts, fresh apricots, peaches, apples, bananas, persimmons, pears, plums, prunes, dates, figs, berries, watermelon.	you get hungry in the afternoon, have a dish of shredded, raw carrots mixed with raisins.	contains many minerals, in varying amounts, needed for healthy development.
Grain Products, Whole or Enriched . . . bread, cereals, crackers, pastas (macaroni, spaghetti, noodles), rice, tortillas, wheat germ.	3 servings each day; same for breast feeding. One slice of bread is one serving. A half-cup of rice, hot cereal, or cooked pasta, 2 corn tortillas, 1 large flour tortilla, a muffin, biscuit, dumpling, pancake, waffle, a 2-inch square of cornbread, and ¾ cup of ready-to-eat cereal (not sugared kind). Each of above makes one serving.	Good source of Vitamin B-1, which helps give your body energy by making sure it uses the various sugars in the food you eat. Iron enrichment helps make hemoglobin, the red substance in blood which carries oxygen to the cells.

Source: Reprinted through the courtesy of the March of Dimes Birth Defects Foundation.

If you begin pregnancy underweight, according to your doctor, or if you weigh less than 120 pounds and gain less than 10 pounds by your twentieth week, you should discuss the matter with your physician.

If you want nutritional expertise, don't rely on your nearest health food store. Ask your medical team for a referral; if this ruffles professional feathers, speak with the nutritionist or dietician at your nearest medical center with maternity facilities. March of Dimes local chapters also can supply information, as can the American College of Obstetricians and Gynecologists, whose address is listed on page 217.

In dealing with your medical team it is wise to be as honest as possible. Your weight is being watched for very sound reasons. Physicians are alert to any sudden jump in weight, because it might be a warning of a complication. This is different from a constant weight gain. If you know that a jump of seven pounds in the month between prenatal visits was due to overeating binges, say so. You'll spare yourself and your physician a genuine worry.

Because of the national interest in nutrition, of changes in rules within the obstetrical world and of the weighty subject of weight gain during pregnancy, here are some specifics that may be of interest or importance to you:

Vitamins. Since proper vitamin intake is extremely important during pregnancy, a good food intake plan such as the one on pages 123–25 should give you what you need.

Many experts say that widely prescribed prenatal vitamins are a matter more of obstetrical habit than of actual need. These vitamins are heavily advertised in publications aimed at doctors. If your doctor strongly believes that you should use these vitamins, please remember that you should think of them as supplements, not substitutes to eating well. You can't skip meals and pop vitamin pills—it just doesn't work that way.

Regarding massive doses of vitamins, which is a current habit for many people, you should avoid this practice during pregnancy. The vitamins that you can tolerate comfortably may harm your baby. According to Dr. Roy Pitkin, former chairman of the ACOG Committee on Nutrition, high doses of Vitamin A during pregnancy may be related to congenital malformation. Vitamin C is concentrated in the fetus, so that high doses may interfere with fetal metabolism. And because a baby may, in fetal life, gear up to eliminate high doses of Vitamin C, after birth the baby may use up its own needed supply of Vitamin C along with the excess Vitamin C, and develop scurvy. Vitamin allowances for pregnancy are very carefully watched and updated by the National Academy of Sciences, and modifications reflect the latest research. The message is, even if you believe very strongly in the value of vitamins, it is best to be guided by medical recommendations during pregnancy.

Iron. Although supplemental vitamins are open to question, supplemental iron as prescribed by your doctor is a *must* during pregnancy and the immediate postpartum months. Your physician may also prescribe supplemental folic acid. (If you have other young children, you should remember to keep your iron pills away from them.) You need iron because your body can't meet the enormous iron demands of pregnancy, and dietary sources aren't sufficient.

Salt. For many, many years salt restriction and diuretics were a routine part of pregnancy. Today, routine salt control is not advised, because sodium serves certain pregnancy needs. Keep up your usual salt intake—using iodized salt—unless there is a definite reason for restriction. As for diuretics, they are no longer considered safe.

Food Additives. You are pregnant in the saccharin/cyclamate era, when there are more than 1,300 officially approved food additives, when newspapers and telecasts daily report that one or another preservative or food coloring can cause cancer, birth defects or a change in the genes that may destine future generations for serious ills.

What should you do? The questions about food additives are many, but the answers vague. The best advice would appear to be that if you have read that a substance is suspect—mutagenic or teratogenic—you may be better off avoiding it even though there is only scant evidence from preliminary laboratory studies. Realizing that your physician may not be supplied with exact answers, you can at least discuss your doubts. There are enough known dangers—alcohol and drugs, for example—against which you can take positive action. It may be more worth your while to eliminate a known problem, such as cigarettes, than to expend effort worrying about a particular food additive.

Some food components do call for attention. Caffeine, a stimulent, found in coffee, tea, colas, soft drinks and numerous products such as cold remedies, can cross the "placental barrier" to an unborn child. The question of whether or not caffeine intake is associated with poor pregnancy experience and/or babies with defects in humans, is a matter of fierce debate and conflicting studies. However, experts say that fewer than six cups of coffee a day—the fewer the better—is a prudent practice. It is thought to be important to cut caffeine consumption when one is trying to conceive and in the first trimester when the fetus is highly vulnerable.

Coping with Weight Gain

If you have always been of normal or near-normal weight, coping with weight gain may mean accepting that you are eating well and gaining to help yourself and your baby. Clear your own mind, and tell yourself that your pregnant silhouette is not the same as a fat person's, that the nine months of pregnancy are only temporary.

If you have always kept your normal weight through rigorous control of what you eat, if you began pregnancy at a near-normal weight because you were dieting, or if you began pregnancy overweight, you have a problem. If rigid weight control has been important to you, it may be very difficult to accept the fact that you have to eat and drink such foods as bread and milk. If you have just successfully completed a diet, pregnancy may make your effort seem a waste. If you are overweight at the start of pregnancy, you may feel depressed and hopeless, and may want to diet; but unless your doctor advises it and makes sure that you are eating a balanced diet, a weight-reduction program, the obstetrical world generally agrees, should *not* be part of pregnancy. Crash dieting, of course, is out!

In their excellent book, *Lying-In: A History of Childbirth in America*, Richard and Dorothy Wertz describe what so many pregnant women have experienced but may not have clearly seen—that the ritual of weighing-in at prenatal visits can be a form of patient obedience training with its concomitant reward or punishment. A good patient follows orders, gains according to schedule and is praised, whereas a woman who gains too much is called everything from gluttonous to irresponsible, and is predicted to have all kinds of complications. Being accountable at the scale certainly can make a woman upset and defensive.

Obstetrician Clark Gillespie, author of a recent book about pregnancy and childbirth, suggests that a woman who gains too much weight try to distract her doctor from a lecture by tears or by bringing him cookies or whatever put the extra weight on her. Neither is a solution, and both are insulting.

Some of the attitudes about weight gain are a carry-over from the days when weight was restricted as a means of preventing toxemia. This turned out to be erroneous. There no longer is the same medical necessity for restricting weight gain; it is the woman who gains too little, in terms of necessary gain, who is the genuine obstetrical worry.

For some women there can be a tendency to relax controls and eat for two—or three—or four. Food can be a way of feeding the inner self at times of stress. It can also symbolize the fact that a baby is really there in the early months of pregnancy when pregnancy is confirmed but there is no visible proof.

If you are having trouble coping, help is available through commercial or informal mutual-support weight-control groups. You can become a member of Weight Watchers with the approval of your physician, who can easily amend or add to the basic food plan. This is a way to have friendly support, to learn new patterns of eating behavior and to help you take weight off after your baby is born. But it does mean getting on a scale.

Weight Watcher groups are led by a person who has successfully lost weight and maintained that loss for a period of time. We questioned a group leader who helped people lose weight while she was pregnant! "It was great," she said. "Women were really impressed by the fact that I could look and dress well. That I wasn't a person with a disease. I was just pregnant. I had been fat all of my life from childhood, and when I was twenty-six I finally lost my weight. For once in my life I was a normal weight after losing forty pounds. Then my husband and I decided to have a child. He was one hundred percent sure, but I was only eighty percent sure of wanting a child, because I was afraid that I would be fat again. My doctors allowed me to follow the Weight Watchers plan with additional milk and fat. I have to admit that at times I was hungry even though I was eating well. Near the end of my pregnancy I passed the twenty-seven pound mark, which was what my doctors wanted me to gain (ultimately I gained thirty-two pounds) and that depressed me. But I looked at my arms and legs, and I knew that the weight was my baby. My husband encouraged me by saying, 'You know that everything is okay, and you'll take care of the weight as soon as the baby is born.' "

Many women have the unhappy experience of higher than necessary gain during pregnancy. Some women never completely lose all of that excessive weight before they again become pregnant. For some this chain of events leads to imprisonment in a great deal of unnecessary and unhealthy poundage. Whether it is help from a formal weight group, from a compassionate physician or nurse who knows nutrition, or from a pregnant friend who is fighting the same battle, some form of support may help you through a troublesome time of pregnancy. If an over-eating problem becomes severe during pregnancy, you might think about some form of psychological help, because the pounds that you are adding may be a distress signal.

Adjusting Nutrition to Your Life

Eating patterns are highly individual. The trick during pregnancy is to adapt intake of essential nutrients to your lifestyle, finances, special needs and, even, nutritional beliefs or special religious requirements. If you have a health problem—a milk intolerance or constant nausea at the start of pregnancy—your doctor can help. If cost is a factor, less expensive cuts of meat, milk, legumes, peanut butter and so on can be alternate sources of valuable nutrients at lower cost. A public health department nurse or nutritionist can be a help on this subject. If business lunches are an essential part of your work world, this should present no problem. Said a literary agent who lunches with authors and editors several times a week, "The first time that I ordered a glass of milk in a French restaurant I was really embarrassed, because I hadn't announced that I was pregnant and it didn't show since it was in the early months. 'Oh,' said the male editor with whom I was having lunch, 'you have an ulcer too. Let's both order milk.' "

Most pregnant women interviewed were highly aware of the importance of nutrition, although many were self-taught because their physicians gave only vague directions. Some felt guilty because of a reliance on convenience or "fast" foods. There is a difference between a fast food such as a hamburger, which is nutritious, and junk food such as potato chips or soda pop. A healthy baby grows on substantial nutrients. Occasional junk food doesn't hurt—a diet of it is a mistake.

Because so many people are seeking alternative ways of eating, it is worth mentioning how one woman doing graduate work in nutrition education handled her food needs during pregnancy. Although she was a lacto-ovo vegetarian before pregnancy (which means that milk and eggs were the only animal proteins that she consumed), for nine months she allowed herself the addition of poultry and fish. "I believe that pregnancy is one time in a woman's life when she is supplying nutrients for a child, and everything should revolve around that. Instead of thinking about individual meals, I tried to have good sources of the various nutrients that I needed each day. I made sure to have top-notch protein—eggs, poultry, fish, peanut butter. If I had vegetable protein—lentils or split peas, for example—I mixed them with animal proteins like milk or cheese for maximum benefit. I made sure to include good carbohydrates in the form of whole grain breads or rice. I made sure to have a couple of vegetables each day and at least one fruit. I drank a quart of skim milk. A typical lunch for me was a split-pea burger (mashed split peas, carrots, bran or wheat germ and an egg) topped with melted cheese. I would also have a salad. I did have desserts and ice cream (my weakness) once a week. I gained about thirty-seven pounds, but my pregnancy went very well and I have a wonderful baby."

DRUGS: A MAJOR PROBLEM IN PREGNANCY

If you are contemplating pregnancy, if you suspect that you may be pregnant, if you are already pregnant, the message is the same: Avoid all drugs—prescription or over-the-counter—unless specifically discussed by you and your physician. Use them only for clearly explained, "good" reasons, where the benefit of the drug outweighs possible risk.

The second part of the message is: "Drugs" means the whole spectrum—everything from aspirin to heroin, ointment salves, sprays, hormone creams, vitamins.

The third part of the message is: During pregnancy, don't self-medicate.

The hazards of drugs in pregnancy first gained national attention because of the thalidomide tragedy of the 1960's and the DES story of the 1970's. Without dwelling on these misfortunes, it is possible to learn from them. Thalidomide quickly showed that a particular drug—in this case a tranquilizer—could result in a deformed baby. Experts point out that thalidomide might never have been discovered as a hazard if it had produced a more subtle effect—a pancreatic defect, for example, that may not have been a problem until adult life, when no one would have suspected that a prenatal drug was the cause. However, thalidomide did produce striking, unmistakable, immediate deformities in enough babies to open a new era of caution. DES, the acronym for diethylstilbestrol, a synthetic hormone once widely prescribed to prevent miscarriages, is another case in point. This is a drug (as was thalidomide) that was given in good faith by responsible physicians. But it had dire consequences that showed up in daughters after adolescence. These consequences included a rare form of cancer and genital abnormalities. Together, the thalidomide and DES stories should suggest to you the absolute necessity of avoiding drugs, and should raise your awareness of the fact that even today, and for many years ahead, physicians—including yours—don't know all the ramifications of the drugs they prescribe.

In general, any drug that you take will reach your baby in varying amounts, and what you can tolerate may be an overdose in the unborn. Drugs can produce birth defects, metabolic problems, chemical effects, and depression or a change in the central-nervous-system function. Sex hormones, estrogens and progresterone can cause congenital defects. The DES experience is the most striking example of this. If you even suspect that you are pregnant you should stop taking birth control pills immediately and refuse any kind of hormone pregnancy test.

We aren't suggesting that you avoid needed drugs. Obviously, there are many genuine medical reasons for medication during pregnancy to treat unrelated medical problems or complications of pregnancy. That is why you want good medical care with a physician who is knowledgeable about the use of drugs. If you develop hypertension, for example, you want to be treated by an expert because certain antihypertension drugs can be hazardous to a baby. Fine tuning in the administration of drugs to pregnant women *can* be done by experts; for example, if corticosteroids must be given to a pregnant woman for a certain illness, other medications can be given to newborns to avert problems at birth and in later life.

If you have a serious need for medication during pregnancy, you should be cared for by an expert, or at least have expert consultation. If you have been accustomed to taking drugs before pregnancy, make a list of everything—including over-the-counter remedies, such as aspirin—and show it to your physician. In some hospital prenatal clinics this subject is considered so important that pregnant women are asked to bring in all pill vials and medication bottles!

Particular drugs continue to make headlines and stir controversy. One such is Bendectin, an anti-nausea drug that has been used over a period of years by some 30 million women worldwide. Opponents—including families with children with birth defects—claim that the drug should not be taken in pregnancy and the FDA has proposed a stiff warning label noting that Bendectin should only be used for severe nausea and vomiting when non-prescription drugs have failed. The debate between the FDA, the manufacturer, the public and scientists is not resolved.

If for any reason your physician suggests a medication you can ask about warnings for use during pregnancy. These are usually listed in package inserts when they are available to the public, which is not always the case. However, your physician—and your library—has reference books that clearly state whatever facts are known about medications on the market. As of 1980, the FDA has required all prescription drugs to be rated according to possible reproductive risk.

You may discover that your physician is more eager for you to avoid drugs than you are. If you have been used to taking a pill to help you sleep, or if you keep aspirin in your office desk drawer, or if you just refill an old prescription for a drug that takes care of diarrhea, it may seem ridiculous or unfair to think that the injunctions against drugs apply to you.

A law student in Seattle described her feeling: "It embarrasses me to tell this story, but in the very early part of my pregnancy I was so jittery and so overwhelmed by the reality of how my life would change that I was very tearful. I remember stopping my car one day in the rain when I couldn't stand the tension any more. I called my obstetrician and said, 'Please, can't you give me a mild tranquilizer just for a short time?' I literally begged him. I was crying, right there in that rain. Of course, he said no and explained why. Eventually I got over my uproar, and my pregnancy became something that I could handle. But I did feel that it was unfair and cruel that I couldn't get any relief when I really needed it."

Tranquilizers are widely prescribed for women, but in pregnancy tranquilizers are out, as your doctor should tell you. Yoga, meditation and sports are alternative ways of relieving tension safely.

Since an estimated 90 percent of women *do* take some form of drugs during pregnancy, it may be useful to have some idea of the problems that different kinds of drugs can cause. This is only a partial listing compiled to show the variety of drugs that can cause problems.

DRUG	EFFECT ON FETUS, BABY OR CHILD
Tetracycline	teeth stains
Streptomycin	hearing loss
Iodine-containing cough medicine	thyroid gland enlargement
Estrogens	heart defects
Androgenic steroids	enlarged clitoris
Aspirin	blood problems
Barbiturates	respiratory depression
Anticoagulants	hemorrhage, facial defects

Drugs are medicinal, or mood- or mind-changing. Whether or not you are in the "drug scene," hard or soft, you should know that a baby born to a narcotic-addicted mother experiences extreme withdrawal symptoms and convulsions and may die; the baby born to a woman who uses amphetamines may have a congenital heart defect. LSD retards fetal growth and can do chromosomal damage. Even methadone can produce severe withdrawal symptoms in frail newborns.

As for marijuana—our interviews with pregnant women show that it is being used during pregnancy and by women concerned with the safety of their babies. Indeed, one woman interviewed grew her own marijuana during pregnancy to assure an uncontaminated supply. However, according to experts, marijuana is not for use during pregnancy and there is a great deal of evidence about the hazards of hard-core drugs.

ALCOHOL: A HAZARD DURING PREGNANCY

This book is designed to inform and promote a better pregnancy for you—not to pry in your personal life. However, there are an estimated one million American women of childbearing age who are alcoholics, and untold numbers of women who are social or weekend drinkers. You know your habits best. But what you may not know is that drinking during pregnancy is dangerous. Says the March of Dimes, "There is no longer any doubt that a woman who drinks heavily during pregnancy runs an increased risk of having children with birth defects. Studies show that many children born to mothers who drank excessively while pregnant have a pattern of physical and mental defects called 'fetal alcohol syndrome.' " Defects include severe growth deficiency, heart defects and malformations. Some scientists believe that alcoholism in pregnancy is the third most common cause of mental retardation.

Alcohol passes directly through the placenta to your baby, and it can do great harm. While the hazards for a heavy drinker—for example, seven glasses a day—are absolutely established, the dangers of lower levels of drinking aren't clear. Many obstetricians consider a glass of wine or so harmless. The March of Dimes, which has supported research on this subject, says, "An occasional drink during pregnancy may not harm your baby. But no one knows how much alcohol is too much . . . the wisest choice is to avoid beer, wine, and hard liquors during pregnancy." Studies question the safety of even moderate drinking, not to mention binge drinking on weekends.

If you drink regularly, be honest and try to seek help, if not from your physician, from the many community resources available—at least for these nine crucial months.

If drinking is a take-it-or-leave-it matter with you, leave it during pregnancy. If a three-martini lunch is part of your working world, you can pass. "Don't let anyone else pressure you," says the literary agent quoted earlier who ordered milk at business lunches.

CIGARETTE SMOKING: GOOD REASONS TO STOP

If you are a cigarette smoker and this is a repeat pregnancy, you may be surprised. This time around, a far stronger effort will be made to convince you to quit. Although evidence has slowly accumulated for several years, it has only been since the late seventies that the case against cigarette smoking during pregnancy has been considered so firm that a national program has begun through the federal government, private health agencies and professional medical groups. This is a worldwide move.

Everyone has heard seemingly everything about the dangers of cigarettes. This is no longer a glamour issue that grabs the spotlight or headlines. There is resistance. There are groups advocating smokers' rights. You don't have to resolve the tobacco controversy during your pregnancy, but for nine months there are two very good reasons for you to quit: If you are a cigarette smoker, you are twice as likely to have a low-birth-weight baby; and if you are a cigarette smoker, you have a greater risk of miscarriage, or later in pregnancy, of stillbirth.

Risk factors of cigarette smoking during pregnancy have been very widely researched, both by following the birth experiences of large groups of women and by laboratory studies. However you feel about your freedom to smoke cigarettes, this is a special matter for your attention during pregnancy.

No one says that it will be easy to give up cigarettes, although for some people it is. It may be particularly difficult for women because of the seductive advertising campaigns aimed directly at them.

If you want to take a very positive action and give up cigarette smoking, at least for the duration of your pregnancy, you will be encouraged to know that there are an estimated 30 million American adults who have quit.

Though the majority of people who give up cigarettes do so unaided, there is plenty of help available. Since you have an immediate need, you might want direct help. It is a plus on your side that smoking withdrawal programs have their greatest success rate in the short term. That is, people who enroll do manage to quit by the end of the program and stay off cigarettes for several months. Since that is your immediate goal, a smoking withdrawal program may be for you.

There are four basic approaches used in smoking cessation programs:

1. *Educational programs,* such as the American Cancer Society Stop Smoking Clinic, Smokenders and the Five Day Plan sponsored by the Seventh Day Adventist Church
2. *Psychotherapy,* including such approaches as hypnosis or group therapy using dramatic role-playing
3. *Behavior modification,* which employs techniques that aren't terrific for pregnancy—electric shock, rapid smoking to cause smoke aversion, and so on
4. *Drug programs* that use agents to simulate the effects of nicotine—also not ideal for pregnant women

Quitting is something to work on in a manner most comfortable for you.

To make it easier for you, you might consider the following:

● Keep cigarette smoking a medical—not a moral—issue. That you are trying to give up cigarettes is not a test of you as a mother, good or bad.

- Make sure that your husband helps. If he is a smoker, you can encourage each other by quitting together.

- Seek out all nonsmoking areas wherever you go. They are very common and a help. Never be embarrassed about giving up cigarettes. Nonsmokers are increasingly chic.

One of the biggest obstacles to giving up cigarettes for women is the fear of weight gain. It is true that once your taste buds are freed of the numbness caused by smoking, food may taste better. If you are eating well during pregnancy, a supply of celery or carrots or the use of cinnamon sticks to chew on can help you over the hurdle without added problems.

If you can give up cigarettes during pregnancy, congratulate yourself. If you absolutely can't and the effort is increasing tension, cut down. Cigarette smoking is dose-related, which means the more you smoke, the greater the hazard.

THE ENVIRONMENT: THE WORLD WE LIVE IN

For all pregnant women, the prize is a good pregnancy and a healthy baby. If you have proper medical attention, eat well and avoid known hazards, you are doing a great deal to help yourself and your baby. You are applying what is known about the prevention of birth defects to your own personal situation. Low birth weight, for example, is the most common birth defect of all. As we have seen, just one positive action—eliminating cigarette smoking during pregnancy—can help prevent that problem.

Medical science still does not know the true impact of the environment on birth defects. It is believed that defects are reflective of an interaction between heredity and the world around us. Research still has a long way to go. This is extraordinarily difficult research because the technology for testing various substances isn't perfect; there may be different susceptibilities among people. Moreover, a potential environmental danger may threaten industry profits, jobs or a convenience to which we have become accustomed. What can you as a protective, pregnant, prospective mother do about unresolved suspicions about the environment?

- Whenever you become pregnant, check with a reputable source, such as the March of Dimes, to see if there are any new, relevant findings that may be important for you to know. Don't panic at scare headlines that implicate this or that substance. What makes news may be early finds, opinions, distortions or useful information. The emotions that it may stir within you are not useful. It's better to find facts than be needlessly frightened.

- If you work during pregnancy, see the points made about occupational hazards in Chapter One.

- If you have a suspected or known family history of genetic disease, be sure to have special medical advice; see Chapter Two.

- If you are a teen-ager, get expert medical help. A clinic at a large medical center will do, but get help to have a healthy baby. If you are over thirty-five, ask about an amniocentesis and get good medical attention.

- If you are not pregnant, be immunized against rubella (German measles). If you are contemplating pregnancy, continue birth control, be immunized and wait until it is safe for you to conceive. If you are already pregnant, have your physician check your rubella status through a simple blood test.

- If you are of childbearing age, are contemplating pregnancy or are already pregnant, avoid exposure to radiation (X-rays).

- If you are pregnant and own a cat, have a blood test done for toxoplasma antibodies to see if you are immune to toxoplasmosis, a common infection in human beings and warm-blooded animals. If you contact toxoplasmosis during pregnancy, either from your pet cat or by eating raw meat, and you are not immune, a birth defect may result. Your cat can be tested, and there are precautions that you can use. Hence, if you are a feline fancier, be on guard.

- If you are pregnant and contract or have ever had a sexually transmitted disease—gonorrhea, syphilis, herpes simplex virus type 2 (also called genital herpes)—have medical attention. Also, ask your physician about cytomegalovirus, a common infection that seldom causes disease after early life, but that can be a problem for a fetus or newborn.

- If you are pregnant, do what you can to avoid bacterial and viral infections.

- After your pregnancy, if the subject of protection for the unborn interests you, you might consider becoming an advocate for more research support. This is a very complex and important matter that may have national priority someday. There are many questions that have yet to be answered, and they are worth answering. For example, if you have taken birth control pills, how does that influence your pregnancy?

A FINAL POINT

Protecting your health during pregnancy and safeguarding your unborn baby are actions with very obvious benefits. If you do what you can with a sense of accomplishment rather than a feeling of deprivation, you can acquire more control over your pregnancy. It then becomes a matter of doing something out of choice—your well-informed choice—rather than being forced to accept someone else's rules. It is one more way to live pregnancy as a woman in command of her life.

6

THE INNER YOU

- When you look in the mirror do you like what you see?
- Do you feel like the person you were before pregnancy?
- Are you able to express your private worries? Will anyone listen?
- How is pregnancy affecting your relationship with the man in your life?

The emotional content of your pregnancy—your sense of who you are, how you react, the joy that you know, the stress that you may feel—matters.

Traditionally, the emotions of pregnancy have been either ridiculed, attributed to hormones with little scientific explanation, or shrugged off with a comment, such as, "When you become a mother all your fears will evaporate, you'll love it." Even worse than being handed a cliché, some pregnant women who have admitted doubts or anxiety have been accused of being unfeminine, unmotherly or hostile to their unborn child. The world wants happy, content pregnant women—and many are. But if a woman feels otherwise, even for transitory periods of her pregnancy, "it makes people very comfortable," said an East Coast lawyer who finally stopped voicing her worries during her first pregnancy.

For many women, pregnancy is a wonderful time. But

pregnancy is too monumental a life experience to be all sweetheart roses.

It is as important for you to understand what is happening in *your* inner emotional life as it is to know the physical development taking place within your womb. It's worth your attention because what is happening to you now in pregnancy—your ability to stay in control of your life—has a lot to do with how you will handle your future. If you deny your feelings—joy, anxiety, strength or vulnerability—if you force yourself to act as you think you should because of your own ingrained attitudes or the expectations of others, you can block your personal growth while a baby is growing inside you.

Interviews with pregnant women reveal what you may have already suspected: The emotional experience of pregnancy can be a roller coaster of highs and lows, exhilarations and fears. Somehow we all arrive at the same destination—the delivery room—but the journey can spin us around, challenge our courage, and certainly race us away from an old, familiar identity.

Most likely, you are not journeying through pregnancy solo. Probably your husband or lover is in the roller-coaster seat beside you. Your mate is not there just at the start—conception—and at the end—childbirth. Whether or not he "seems interested" or senses the reality of the baby as vividly as you do, your man experiences a range of strong feelings and changes that he may be less able to identify or express than you are.

As a couple, you both undergo new pressure; you have to rely on each other in new ways; extreme change is imminent; you may make unsuspected demands and have expectations of each other that neither you nor your partner can even begin to meet unless you talk about them. You can do a great deal to help yourself—and each other—if you realize there are going to be stresses and strains and that you'll be able to cope with them.

THE ABC'S OF TAKING CARE OF YOU

A. Acknowledge the fact that emotions and feelings are very much part of pregnancy, and that it is better to identify your reactions than to be startled or afraid of them.

B. Find someone with whom you can share your emotions without embarrassment or judgments about your behavior.

C. Select medical care that provides encouragement and support. If any of the emotions of pregnancy trouble you to the extent that your worries or doubts increase in intensity or duration, schedule a special visit to your medical team.

D. Take a look at your life, consider whether there is anything adding to your burdens right now—for example, a shaky marriage, financial insecurity, responsibility for other children with no help—and realize that you may need relief or at least an opportunity to talk about these additional worries.

E. Take a look at your pregnancy so far. Are you continuing to advance along lines that were important to you before pregnancy? Do you have activities and interests that occupy you sufficiently so that you are distracted from always thinking about the baby? If you have stopped working, are you making good use of empty time? Are you acquiring any new skills unrelated to childbearing? In other words—are you still growing as a person?

F. Take a look at your pregnancy, and be honest about obstetrical strain—are you in any kind of high-risk situation or have you had obstetrical problems in the past? If so, you want extra support and encouragement from your medical team.

G. Try to attend *early* prenatal classes that give you an opportunity to learn about pregnancy, and ask questions about the emotional changes you may be experiencing. Do exercises to keep your body in good condition. Learn about newborn care so that you will cope rather than crumble.

H. Think through how you want to deliver your baby—but never put all of your hopes on having an ideal experience. Realize that while labor and delivery are difficult, if you replace fear and anxiety with relaxation techniques and knowledge about how your body will act, childbirth will be better. Do everything you can well in advance to assure yourself of delivery in a warm, supportive atmosphere that gives you a maximum opportunity to be with your mate and new baby. Immediate closeness to your baby may facilitate early mothering.

I. During your pregnancy, explore alternative means of relieving tension. This makes sense, because you are trying to avoid such things as alcohol and tranquilizers. Many pregnant women favor yoga, some use relaxation techniques, others may vent feelings through sports or punching a pillow.

J. Take charge of your ninth month. This is important because many women stop working at this time and feel suddenly bereft. All women become cumbersome, tired of pregnancy and anxious about delivery. This is the time to have engrossing reading material handy when you aren't doing a series of things to make your life easier after the baby arrives. This includes having your hair cut; stocking your larder; freezing a month's worth of dinners; lining up homemaker services or baby sitters. This also is a good time to screen pediatricians.

K. If you know in advance that you will have a cesarean section or wind up having one, contact a local group of parents who have gone through the experience. If there is no local group, use the source on page 219. A cesarean birth is different from vaginal delivery in an emotional as well as a physical sense. These groups can offer empathy and information.

L. However you deliver, as soon as you can, grab someone—even in the hospital—and talk about your whole delivery experience. Literally relive it from start to finish. Unless you express feelings and reactions provoked by childbirth, you can emerge with memories that will fade but can leave you scarred. You want to emerge from childbirth with an intact personality, and this is one simple way to help yourself achieve that by "talking it out."

M. The arrival of a baby is one of the greatest traumas of adult life—there is more and more evidence about this point—and you can help yourself by affiliating for a time with a new parents' group.

N. Postpartum depression can occur. It can be mild or serious. It is no joke. If you are having trouble, get professional help fast.

O.–Z. Finally, do whatever you can to enjoy your pregnancy.

As you can see, support is a vital part of an emotionally healthy pregnancy. When we spotlight some of the stress factors and emotions of pregnancy, this will become especially clear. For example, vulnerability and fear of abandonment are common feelings of pregnant women. With proper support, these feelings can be eased and lessened.

Who, then, should be on your support team—who can be there for you?

YOUR PREGNANCY SUPPORT TEAM

The first person to bolster you has to be you yourself. You have to work at taking care of yourself. Then comes your mate; family members who help rather than hinder; friends you like and trust. If you can find at least one person to listen without judging you, it can be a great comfort. It doesn't matter who this person is. Some pregnant women find it easier to confide in older women they know through work or socially rather than a mother or close relative.

In seeking emotional support, there is a great resource for you—other pregnant women. As Judy Norsigian of the Boston Women's Health Collective, author of *Our Bodies, Ourselves,* said in an interview, "We have been overconditioned to look to the medical professions for assistance. There is often more benefit in getting suppo t and information from others going through a similar experience." Since much of the information in this book derives from pregnant women, we also know that there is great value in shared experiences. You may meet women with whom you have little else in common save pregnancy, and you each may be handling pregnancy differently, but you can help each other by caring and being patient. You both know that there are things pregnant women want to say. Early prenatal classes are an excellent way to set up an informal network of pregnant friends; in some communities there are expectant mothers' talk groups. If you are isolated in the sense that you are working and have little contact with other pregnant women, a physician or midwife may be able to make introductions to other pregnant women in similar positions. You can do a lot by telephone!

Support is a way of making your pregnancy better. We are not trying to suggest that pregnancy is awesome or that you will be severely troubled. We are suggesting support as a means of making pregnancy stress free.

If you discover, however, that you are bothered by strong emotions frequently or with intensity; if you are having trouble sleeping; if you feel somehow unable to cope with the pressures of pregnancy and coming motherhood; or if you are rattled by mood swings, you should speak with your physician.

Doctors are being told that it is more important to listen to their patients than to reach for a prescription pad. More than likely, your physician can be of help. However, some physicians are cold or indifferent to emotional matters; some are poorly trained to help; some are just too busy. If you feel your physician can be of help, schedule a visit just to discuss your feelings.

Many women, however, are unable to speak frankly with their physicians. In one study where more than 81 percent of the women questioned admitted to fears and worries, only 17 percent told their fears to their doctors.

If you discover that you are worried or upset and that neither your support team nor your physician can make a difference, you should seek at least temporary psychological help. It is far better to try to handle a problem during your pregnancy than to go into motherhood with unresolved conflicts or problems. Some psychologists specialize in aiding pregnant women and/or their mates. See the "Resourses to TAP" section of the appendix. If you have no access to this kind of help, you might try arranging a private visit to a hospital social worker or a nurse specialist in maternity. Whether it's through an informal support team or a talk with a physician or psychologist, you can devise means of easing yourself through pregnancy. You may not be able to see the strain factors of pregnancy as clearly as the physical factors, because they are just not publicized. Says Manhattan social worker Tamara Engel, who has professional experience in helping pregnant women, "When I was pregnant in 1974 to 1975 I wanted to read everything I could about the emotional aspects of pregnancy. I went to a bookstore, and the woman said, 'If you want books about stretch marks, I'll give you books about stretch marks. If you are interested in terms of what to expect about your moods or what will happen in your marital relationship, forget it!' " Tamara Engel wound up keeping a diary of her pregnancy to help her cope with her experiences. You might find that a helpful idea for you.

STRESS FACTORS OF PREGNANCY

For pregnant women, change is extraordinary and rapid. In nine months you go from a body that you have known all your life to one distorted and different; you go from being an individual whose identity you know to somebody else—a mother. Pregnancy is a leap into the unknown, and that can be terrifying.

Even a generation ago, pregnancy was simpler because there were role models to identify with and lean on for advice and comfort. Today, you might be having a first child at forty while your friends already are the parents of teen-agers; you may be having a first child in a second marriage; or you may be having a first child at a crucial moment in your career. Though some of us are competent in our own fields, we have no real preparation for pregnancy or motherhood.

Stress does exist in pregnancy. Don't be put off by the word "stress." It refers only to how you adapt to change. Change can be something happy, like pregnancy, or wonderful, like an outstanding personal achievement. On a life-stress scale of 100 (the point of highest stress, the death of a spouse), pregnancy ranks 40, above such other stress categories as mortgage foreclosure and sex problems. Many other stress points—for example, a change of residence, which is 20 points—are a fact of life for many pregnant women as well. The ordinary stress impact of pregnancy has a ripple effect, causing other changes, each one of which adds another burden of tension or conflict.

Emotions and Reactions

No single emotional experience is the same for all pregnant women. But there are some common feelings, anxieties and actions. You may experience some of them—or none—but perhaps one will strike a responsive note within you.

Joy. Most women know about the happiness of being pregnant. In fact, many of the women who allowed interviews for this book did so because they were excited and exultant. But, like many of the emotions you'll experience in these nine months, joy may be transitory. One woman, an art director, told us she had "two really terrific moments. The first was the day that I learned that I was pregnant. The second was eight months later when the special birth announcement I had designed came back from the printer with a blank for the baby's name, birth date and weight."

Joy is there for you, but sometimes there can be barriers to experiencing it. Social worker Patsy Turrini has pointed out that we Americans can have trouble permitting ourselves our feelings of pleasure. We often feel guilty about feeling good. If you want the baby more than your husband does; if you forgot birth control one night in the middle of your ovulatory cycle and that's your secret; if this baby is fulfilling your secret desires, you may not allow yourself to express happy feelings, or you may have trouble showing your joy to others. Perhaps your husband or boss or even a close friend is threatened by your happiness. If so, find someone else or another way to rejoice.

Because of a poor self-image, we may deny ourselves trust or happy anticipation. Writer Phyllis Theroux expressed it this way: "There is something very deep within most of us that checks our earlier impulses to trust life. Upon being told that I was pregnant, for instance, I could not shake the conviction that I would probably give birth to an acorn squash, and it was only when that perfectly beautiful child was held before my eyes that I had faith in what had gone before. So much for my faith. Fortunately, the outcome did not greatly depend on it."

Vulnerability and isolation. Vulnerability—the feeling of being out of control, dependent, susceptible to hurt or afraid that your baby will be hurt—is a condition of pregnancy that can be heightened by feelings of isolation. Women withdraw at periods to perform some of the emotional tasks of pregnancy—for example, to accept the reality of pregnancy in the first trimester when there is no visible belly. Women withdraw, too, because they become wrapped up in themselves and shut other people out. This in turn leads some women to think their pregnancy is different from everyone else's, and if it isn't entirely pleasant they feel vulnerable and alone. Just bear in mind that there is no norm in pregnancy and there is no superwoman.

Anxiety, doubts. According to Dr. Joan Zuckerberg, a New York City clinical psychologist who is part of a special psychological consultation service for parents and prospective parents, "A majority of pregnant women experience considerable separation anxiety in making the psychic transition from single woman to pregnancy to motherhood. This anxiety is often concretized and expressed as a fear of death. Added to this fear is the reality that not that far behind us in time are the generations of women for whom childbirth was life-threatening, and a healthy baby a possibility rather than a probability. Also, the vast majority of American births take place in crisis centers for disease and death—hospitals—and until recently, the medical world looked at normal pregnancy as an illness. For many pregnant women, childbirth may be the first time that they have been hospital patients; some husbands shun being present at delivery because of their own fears of sickness."

Pregnancy is not sickness, but certainly there is a realistic expectation that our bodies will go through trauma. One woman said, "I have never had stitches in my life, and all of a sudden I realized that I would have to have an episiotomy and part of my body would be cut. That freaked me out. I would never be whole and perfect again."

Regarding the fear of death, there is reason to extend the definition of death somewhat for today's pregnant woman. We are speaking now of the "death" of the person you have always been, a change in your identity that may be pressuring you now. It is our contention that this death shouldn't happen if you have an active, satisfying pregnancy that allows you to progress in your interests— if you experience pregnancy as a process leading you to motherhood rather than as a total abandonment of yourself for a new role.

It is not crazy or sick or unreasonable for pregnant women to worry that motherhood will be an end to hard-won personal gains. We are part of an era when women are being valued for their talents and independence as well as for their ability to bear children. But since this is a time of transition, in pregnancy you come smack up against old ideas.

Poet Adrienne Rich described the power of this collision: "As soon as I was visibly and clearly pregnant, I felt for the first time in my adolescent and adult life not guilty. The atmosphere of approval in which I was bathed— even by strangers on the street, it seemed—was like an aura I carried with me, in which doubts, fears, misgivings met with absolute denial: This is what women have always done."

The idea that we achieve nothing—regardless of our solid accomplishments—unless we are mothers still has some hold. Sometimes we can even put an end to ourselves to show our commitment to an unborn child. Poet Rich stopped writing, started sewing and collecting baby clothes. She "blotted out as much as possible the woman I had been a few months earlier." By the time of delivery, she had developed a rash that was later diagnosed as an allergy to pregnancy.

Whether it is an allergy or midnight worry or a compulsive desire to overeat, our personal reactions to pregnancy surface in other ways. It is far better to try to learn what we really feel about this change in our lives, because squelching feelings does not eliminate them.

Although we are not trained psychologists, we can understand that our fears, rather than being enemies, may have important meanings if we are willing to look at them instead of bolting away.

Fear of loss. Despite the fact that most babies are healthy, the fear of a lost or harmed baby is something that all pregnant women—and their mates—live with whether on a conscious level or not. But there are ways of dealing with this fear.

The first is by handling it on a realistic level. You can reassure yourself that you are doing all that you can do to have a healthy pregnancy by having good prenatal care, eating well, remaining active physically and mentally. Your physician or midwife or childbirth educator can also give you the facts—in as much detail as you want—about the safety of childbirth and the probability of a healthy baby.

In some prepared childbirth classes, prospective parents are asked to discuss what would happen in the event of the loss of a baby or of a birth defect. Some couples are totally unable to speak to this point; some individuals have been furious at having the subject mentioned. It is too frightening for them to handle. Being afraid to look at a subject can make it worse.

If you can quietly ask yourself, "What would I do if . . . ?" and fill in your worst fear, you may at least gain some sense of mastery over fate and your future rather than remain a passive potential victim. Although the chances of a problem are remote, it is useful to know that if a loss or defect occurs, there are other parents who have gone through the same thing (who can be reached through childbirth educators or medical professionals) who may be of genuine help and emotional comfort.

Ambivalence. Less severe than fear of tragedy, but no less plaguing to you, may be a shifting sense of ambivalence about your pregnancy. Even if yours is a wanted pregnancy, it is natural to feel doubts. One of the most candid women interviewed for this book said she was still ambivalent when she was awaiting childbirth five days past her due date.

Ambivalence is understandable in view of the kind of change that you are undergoing. The physical aspect of pregnancy can well symbolize what has to occur in your psyche. If you think about it, you will realize that your baby is really a foreign invader and your body is geared, through its immune system, to fight off invaders. Even though your baby is a stranger, made up of your genes and your mate's, it is allowed to incubate peacefully within your body thanks to a tissue called the trophoblast, which protects and nourishes it. The psyche also enables us to accept and nurture another being, identify it as ours, and then let go at the end of nine months. This psychic process works through dreams and fantasy, odd behavior, hostility, happiness and other ways science has only begun to chart. If you understand that your reactions—including ambivalence—may represent a way of adjusting to a new role, they may seem less peculiar.

Change in Body Image

Your growing body is such an obvious and predictable aspect of your pregnancy that it might not seem necessary to point out how the experience of continual body change can influence the inner you. However, your body image—the way that you perceive yourself, your understanding of the space that you occupy, your sense of where you end and the rest of the world begins—is part of your essential self-identity. Body image is one of the ways that you know that "this is me, this is who I am." Pregnancy disrupts that familiar sense of body image. This can be unsettling because, as Janie Spelton Weinberg, a nursing instructor at the University of Connecticut, has written, "a distortion of customary body image is experienced as a distortion of self."

Research into body-image change during pregnancy has shown that your perception of your size will increase as your pregnancy progresses. This seems altogether natural and proper and may represent another way of adapting emotionally to impending motherhood. However, research done by Dr. Jacqueline Fawcett, an assistant professor of nursing at the University of Connecticut, shows that immediately after childbirth your perception of your body size may be different from reality. You may "see" yourself as being smaller than you are. By two months after childbirth this false perception may be adjusted. However, the time between childbirth and two months postpartum is an emotionally vulnerable one. The realization that you are not as slim as you thought despite giving birth may cause you dismay and disappointment when you need those feelings least.

How do you deal with body image change during pregnancy and postpartum? There are several ways. First, it helps to acknowledge the fact that having a changing body can by itself be a very unsettling experience. You can grasp some of the changes by studying the drawings of pregnant women in books like *Our Bodies, Ourselves*. That kind of homework can help prepare you for what you will look like in the months ahead. Also, seek good things to think and say about your body during pregnancy. This is something you may have to do for yourself, because pregnancy does not have a high glamour rating. Finally, you can attend maternal exercise classes during pregnancy to keep your body in shape and to know that you are in control even if your body looks different.

To avoid postpartum letdown, ask your physician or nurse or a woman you trust who has had a baby recently to give you an *honest* assessment of how long it will take you to get back into reasonable shape. In your ninth month (or before), read about postpartum exercises, and if you can, sign up for exercise classes beginning after the baby is born.

Body image change is part of pregnancy. If you are prepared, you will feel better about yourself, and you will have the comfort and reassurance of knowing that a return to your normal self will be entirely possible, no matter how huge and ungainly you become. Remember, it's not forever.

The Influence of Your Mother on Your Pregnancy

In addition to the physical, social, economic and emotional burdens of becoming a mother, something else takes place. Pregnancy is a time when you come up against your past memories of your mother, particularly of how she reacted to pregnancy and childrearing. You also have to interact with your mother in a new way. You are no longer just a daughter; you are in the process of matching her in the game of motherhood. You are also going to produce a grandchild.

If your mother had a bad obstetrical experience, one that she talked about since your childhood, you may fear childbirth. If she really wasn't keen on being a mother, this may influence how you think of your new role. The important thing for you to keep in mind is this: Your pregnancy is unique and separate. You are not reliving your mother's experience. And as a mother, you will be creating a brand-new child/mother relationship.

If you and your mother have been in conscious or subtle competition, watch out during pregnancy. You may find yourself trying to outdo her. This attempt can take bizarre forms. For example, one woman we interviewed developed a whole variety of aches and complaints to make herself conspicuous in her "suffering" during pregnancy. Her own mother was proud of the fact that she sailed through pregnancy. By suffering, her daughter showed that she was different from her mother.

Many of us want attention from our mothers during pregnancy, and some of us receive affection and happy support. However, don't start by expecting too much, because your mother is having her own reactions to becoming a grandmother. Also, some mothers are unable to give. Nonetheless we do need a form of "mothering" during pregnancy. Your support team can provide an adult version of the kind of attention and concern the child in all of us craves.

You may help yourself as well if you realize that some women see childbearing as a way of pleasing or giving a special gift—a grandchild—to their mothers. Try to avoid that scene. Pregnancy is not a command performance, and your baby belongs to you and your mate.

Also, if the ideas in this book are in tempo with your own, you may live a pregnancy vastly different from your mother's. This can lead to a negative reaction on her part. You may at some point have to say what one twenty-two-year-old administrative assistant said: "Ma, leave me alone. I am going to work until the day I deliver. I have to live my life."

Your Mate and Your Relationship

When you become pregnant, you enter that state with attitudes and anticipations out of sync with reality. So does your mate. Said a thirty-five-year-old expectant father, "I've always associated pregnancy with something special and mysterious. I am very disillusioned and disappointed. It's just another part of living."

A corporate executive said, "I thought that pregnancy would be a matter for my wife; that I would just ask her how she was doing after each visit to her doctor. Instead, I feel incredibly tense and pressured. My health has been terrible. I have even gone to my doctor for a check-up. He says that I am reacting to pregnancy, and there is nothing wrong with me."

And a news photographer said, "My mother nearly died giving birth to me—or so she has told me all of my life. I am more frightened of this experience than my wife is. Actually it's been *very* positive."

The male experience of pregnancy is very real and extremely important. Unfortunately, more is known about your emotions and reactions than your husband's. One area has been explored and widely publicized—the feelings of men who have participated in the delivery of their child—but the truth of the matter is that men live the *whole* pregnancy experience.

The very psychological journey you are making—the transit from one identity to an altered one, the confrontation with influences from your past, the fear of the future and the unknown—is being made by the man in your life too. Equally important, as a couple you are progressing through time towards parenthood, passing a lot of stress points along the way.

If you have some insight into the male experience of pregnancy, if you at least recognize some of the pressures on your mate, if both of you think the stress factors are affecting you as a couple, you may be better able to emerge as a new family than as two people somewhat alienated, resentful and suddenly parents.

Just as you are pregnant at a time when life for a woman has drastically changed, your husband is an expectant father at a time when a new image of fatherhood is beginning to emerge. Look around at the new fathers wearing babies in pouches on their chests or carrying toddlers in backpacks; think of the stories you have read about men who have said that being present for the delivery of their child was one of life's greatest experiences. Men are in delivery rooms all over America—men of all different ages and backgrounds—and that would not be happening if there wasn't a desire to share in the moment of birth and a deep resentment against the tradition of expectant fathers as forgotten men.

Expectant fathers who participate—the ones who happily attend prepared childbirth classes and who are supportive throughout pregnancy—are heroes of the New Masculinity, a male identity in which it is all right to nurture and be tender without losing male pride.

You may very much want your mate to be that kind of expectant father—and both of you can suffer if he isn't ready for the role or interested in it. Just as the modern pregnancy experience is allowing you to be what you want to be, you have to allow your mate equal freedom. Rather than try to force stereotypes or ideals on an unwilling man, it's better to have an understanding of some of the male reactions to pregnancy and how they may be disguised in your daily lives together.

Interviews for this book confirm what one team of researchers at the Tucson Medical Center reported in *Maternal Child Nursing:* "Fathers do respond quite dramatically to their mates' emotional changes and demands . . . physiological changes, and . . . altered body image. What's more, they experience their own inward changes."

One of the most striking changes centers on an intensification of the traditional role of man as provider and breadwinner. Even if you are a working pregnant woman who plans to be a working mother, your husband will feel a new demand to be the support of his family. Even if you both have planned for you to stop working—a decision that your husband approves and wants—your husband may be reeling from a new burden of financial responsibility. The value of a woman's income does not hit home until the reality of pregnancy may remove that income. Many male worries about the welfare of the pregnant mate may be masked by a concern for money and expenses. In our culture, that's an appropriate way for a strong man to express concern and inner uncertainty.

Because it is a practical concern, this is one area that can be discussed. Other concerns may never be actually expressed by your mate, but may show up in his actions. One pregnant woman who was particularly eager to discuss what was happening in her marriage during her second pregnancy had this to say: "About the end of my seventh month, things became so bad that I thought that our marriage was over. I am a fairly decent housekeeper and cook. My husband never had criticized me before. Then, night after night, as soon as he came home from work, he began to list everything wrong in the house; he hated everything I put on the table. Our little boy could do nothing right. There was constant shouting. At first, I just couldn't understand what was happening. After all, we had been through pregnancy before, and it was a fine time for both of us. Finally I cornered him and made him talk to me. He admitted that he was scared by the responsibility of having a second child, that that really made him a father. He felt that he was old and his life was over."

Some men are able to articulate their concerns. Said a Detroit salesman whose wife is pregnant for the first time, "I have four worries: One, will I always be able to make a living? Two, will I be a good father? Three, can I avoid being jealous of my own kid? Four, how is my life going to change?"

Your husband's reactions to you are, of course, enormously important. They can vary from enthusiasm and joy to seeming indifference or even cruelty. But you must remember your husband is under new stress, just as you are. Try to talk things out. After all, you have a joint investment here!

DEFUSING COUPLE STRESS DURING PREGNANCY

The most powerful weapons you have to combat couple stress during pregnancy are your love for each other, your mutual desire for a child and your ability to communicate. Even if your love relationship isn't perfect, even if one of you wants a baby more than the other, the ability to communicate can prevent some problems and solve others.

It is familiar advice to say that you have to talk to each other about your thoughts, but in pregnancy there is a subtle difference. This time you have to uncover and identify just what it is you really expect of each other during these nine months, the childbirth and the early months with your new baby.

For example, you may be deluding yourself that your husband or lover really wants or intends to be with you during labor. If you can be honest together, you can find a substitute support person. You and your mate will have honored your feelings and rights. You may resent his decision, but at least you won't have to cope with a man who doesn't want to be there when you are in labor.

As you and your mate discuss your feelings during these nine months, you both can expect some hidden attitudes that might shock you. For example, one man was so aghast when his wife told him of her ambivalent feelings about childbearing that he decided that she was "abnormal or sick, because women are supposed to be happy." If you can speak with each other comfortably, even when hurtful attitudes emerge, you can deal with them.

If you and your mate can attend early childbirth classes together, he may be better able to understand and share the whole pregnancy experience.

If you can work out a pregnancy "contract"—and a plan for early child care—everyone may be stronger. According to childbirth educator Cherry Wunderlich of Washington, D.C., who has reviewed much of the research on the father's experience of pregnancy, a study by R. A. Fein indicates that "things go better if there are definite role assignments, whatever they are." This means deciding who does what. You may opt for a traditional setup: woman as childbearer and homemaker, husband as weekend father. If bottle-feeding, you may decide that you will alternate night feedings, and each will have weekend time off. It's the realistic, reasonable contract— worked out in advance—that is important. It can always be amended later.

Other ways to relieve couple stress during pregnancy include a mutual assessment of your new financial structure. If you plan to continue working, there will be crucial decisions about the cost of child care. You can relieve your husband's anxieties about finances by participating in solutions. Thus you can offer proof that he is not all alone with heavy responsibility.

While this nation has made progress in allowing working pregnant women to take maternity leaves, we are still in the dark ages regarding time off for new fathers. Although there is substantial evidence that immediate close contact and involvement with an infant are essential to the strength and growth of a family, your husband will not be able to spend time with you and your new baby unless you plan strategy and arguments to use with his employer. It is well understood that a man must take time off on the day of delivery, but it is not well understood that a new father needs other leave time as well.

In a major company, when one new father wanted to take a week off to help care for a premature newborn, his employer offered to hire a nurse and pay all expenses if the young man would go on a planned sales trip. The young man went on the trip, but refused the bribe, because he did not want to build up "debts" that would make him owe his company a favor. In the same company, another new father had made it clear early in the months of his wife's pregnancy that he expected leave time. He got it and offers this advice: "If you stand up for what you believe, educate your employer, they will go along with what you want."

If you have worked during your pregnancy, you will be familiar with the strategy and arguments that your mate can adapt for use with his employer when your baby is born and during the childrearing years ahead. Ideally, you should start to arrange things early, so that if a child becomes sick the mother *or* father can take the necessary time off.

THE EMOTIONAL ROLLER COASTER: IS IT WORTH IT?

Your baby is, of course, the supreme reward of pregnancy. However, your nine-month experience of changing emotions and relationships has a personal bonus for you as well. If, during pregnancy, you actively work at taking care of yourself and learn to know your own feelings and reactions better; if you learn to value your own instincts and emotions and listen to yourself; if you learn to find and benefit from having others you trust, you will have taken another giant step forward. If your pregnancy offers an opportunity for you and your mate to know each other better, your lives will be richer. Even though you may have been on an emotional roller coaster, you will have arrived at your destination on your feet. You can be very proud of yourself for that. It is great to live proud!

7

THE OUTER YOU: LOOKING GOOD

The way you look during pregnancy telegraphs the way you feel, and the image you convey will be the key in determining how others respond to you.

If your clothing is neat and stylish, your face and hair properly groomed and your bearing confident, you will feel good and in turn will convey the message that your pregnancy does not indicate either a withdrawal from your normal activities or a cessation in your commitment to your job.

You cannot hide your belly. Don't apologize for your pregnancy by trying to camouflage your figure. It implies that you are uncertain about yourself and your pregnancy, and may cause others to think you have a lack of self-respect and confidence about your impending role. Be proud of your condition, and dress to make yourself as attractive as possible.

Lester Hayatt, one of the United States' leading maternity designers, characterized his clothing as "picker-uppers." He said, "Clothes make you feel better. That's normal for everyone, pregnant or not. But it's even more important in pregnancy because you *do* have a figure problem and are even more conscious of the way you look."

We know that society long characterized pregnant women as weak and unsightly, and the accepted behavior was to stay out of sight during much of the nine months. Even with the changing times, many people are still uncomfortable in the company of a pregnant woman.

It is up to you to change this perception, and one of the easiest ways to do it is by dressing well. A fourth-grade teacher from Wisconsin told us that "people tend to stereotype pregnant women as haggard and unattractive, but it's not necessary to confirm that image." Clothing can help dispel some of these old myths, can help create a positive image for you and can lend credence to the verbal commitment you have given to your employer about your future work plans. You will be showing that you are proud of your pregnancy and confident of yourself through your dress and your demeanor.

"It's hard to look great with a sixty-inch waist," said one office manager, "but my husband insisted that I buy very fashionable maternity clothes. I finally did, and what a difference it made. I loved my clothing and I loved being pregnant. Not only did I look terrific, but I felt great, and ultimately my office forgot that I was pregnant."

DRESSING FOR AN ACTIVE PREGNANCY

The way you live during your pregnancy is completely different from the way pregnant women lived only a few years ago. Whether you work or not, you are active. Pregnancy does not indicate isolation.

You are out—whether it is at work, on the tennis courts, or at an elegant restaurant. You want to look smashing, have a few things to carry you through your pregnancy and invest wisely on your maternity wardrobe.

When you become pregnant, you shouldn't have to give up the styles you followed in ready-to-wear clothing, but you may be surprised to learn that fashionable maternity clothing is limited. One reason for this is that until recently there was not a large-enough market for stylish maternity clothes. Women stayed home during their pregnancies. They did not work, nor were they usually active, so there was no need for a variety of maternity clothes. Inexpensive cotton tops with puffed sleeves, a ruffled neckline and cotton skirts and pants were what was offered and what was purchased.

Another reason was the pregnant woman herself. In fact, you may be a little at fault yourself if you agree with two arguments that have persisted about maternity clothes through the years: (1) "It's only for a short period of time, so I don't want to spend the money," and (2) "The quality of the clothing is not very good, so I won't buy anything."

If you think about these statements, however, you may want to reconsider the arguments. For one thing, you will be wearing maternity clothing for six months—or half a year. This usually spans at least one season, possibly more. You would purchase some new clothing to keep up with current fashions anyway, even if you were not pregnant. Since clothing has a limited lifespan, maternity clothing will just replace normal seasonal purchases.

Regarding the quality of the clothing, you *do* have some justification in the criticism. The fabric for maternity clothing is not of as high a quality as standard ready-to-wear clothing. But you are not paying the same prices either, nor are you purchasing this clothing for a long-term investment. You are buying it just as you would a few fill-in pieces each season, to keep up with the styles and to modify your appearance to accommodate your changing figure.

Yet it is often difficult to find maternity clothing that is both stylish and wearable. As one teacher said, "One of the biggest problems I had was finding clothes that looked reasonably professional. They have all those beautiful little sundresses that you can whip around your terrace in and entertain in—but you can't exactly convey a professional image with them."

The maternity clothes market is inconsistent. There are some high-fashion maternity boutiques, there are some department stores that carry wonderful maternity clothes, but more often than not the maternity clothes available today are largely those that women have been accustomed to in the past. Maternity wear has not kept up with the active pregnant woman today.

Scouting the Market

One way to find the maternity clothing that you want to wear is to scout the market. As soon as you become pregnant, set aside a day and case the maternity clothes shops in your community. It is not necessary—and probably not advisable—to buy anything at this point. You may have to do a little basic research and take some time and effort to find maternity clothing suitable for you, but if you are really interested you will find it.

If you live in a large city, there is probably at least one maternity boutique in town. Even if it is on the other side of town, make a trip to see what is available. Explain to the salesperson what kind of life you expect to lead over the next few months, and tell her what kind of budget you have. Look around to get an indication of what is available, and ask what will be coming in within the next few months.

Look around for other pregnant women and ask anyone wearing clothing you particularly like where she bought it. Then track down the store. Pregnant women love to share—especially when it involves looking good with a protruding belly.

The yellow pages may also have a listing of the maternity stores in your area. You can save a little footwork by calling and asking whether they carry upbeat or traditional maternity clothing. Most will answer honestly, and you can eliminate those that do not carry what you want.

You may also find a discount maternity outlet in your area. They may not have the type of fashionable clothing you desire, but it will help you learn what is available and will provide a basis for comparison.

You may even be able to locate a maternity resale boutique. This is a store where women who have been pregnant sell their clothing to other pregnant women at second-hand prices. Check carefully, because the prices may be just as competitive and the clothing somewhat worn. On the other hand, you may find some terrific buys.

If you live in a small town, a little creative pursuit may be necessary. You may even want to make a trip to the nearest large city to check out a major department store. Call the store ahead of time, speak to the maternity department and ask what type of clothing they carry. Ask if they have a brochure, and request that one be sent to you. You may be able to purchase your things via mail.

Most salespeople will be delighted to talk to you on the telephone, because it may mean a sale for them. Explain what you want and the type of clothing you like, and tell that person what you think you will need. Ask if they would be willing to send you a few items. If you have a charge account at the store, charge your purchases. If not, ask the price, including mailing charges, and send a check. You can usually get a refund if the merchandise you return has not been worn and the merchandise tags are still on it.

You may want to consider making your own maternity clothing. There are many fashionable maternity patterns now on the market and you will get a great deal of pleasure from making your own things tailored to your own needs and desires.

If you do not sew, you may want to look around for someone who does and hire that person to make you a few things. You probably will not save any money (because aside from buying the patterns and fabrics you will have to pay the seamstress for her time), but you will have maternity clothing that you will love wearing.

During your scouting trip you will probably discover that the type and quality of maternity clothes vary tremendously from store to store and community to community. Some specialty stores have a wonderful selection of apparel, some department stores may not even have a maternity department. If they do, they may be run by salespeople like the buyer at one of New England's largest department stores who said, "I really can't talk about maternity fashions because I've never been pregnant myself." This woman is deciding what type of maternity clothing will be available to you!

What You Can Do to Demand Better Maternity Clothing

Until recently there was not a broad enough demand for stylish, active maternity clothes. Manufacturers made clothing that had the widest appeal, and store buyers stocked their maternity departments with "supermarket clothing," those traditional styles that the greatest number of women would buy.

You *do* have some clout in this area. Speak up. Tell the buyer in your local store that you are dissatisfied with the clothing available. Tell her why and what you would like. Maternity buyers usually buy three months ahead of the season, so there is time for your local buyer to stock some stylish clothing in your local store. This is also why a scouting trip can be important for you.

If you are really serious, write a letter to the store's marketing and merchandising vice-president. Tell him or her that you are dissatisfied with the maternity selections available, and suggest that a more fashionable look might bring the store more customers. Ask for what you want. Others have—and it is reflected in the maternity boutiques and department stores that carry stylish maternity clothing and active sportswear. Look for it, ask for it, and you will find it.

Maternity Don'ts

One of the things that many women do—and that we are going to discourage—is to wear regular clothing two sizes larger than they would normally. This is not a good idea for several reasons:

- The clothing will be larger in the shoulders and will look oversized. Maternity clothes are cut differently, with more of a triangle shape, smaller on top, wider through the back and bustline and larger in the belly.

- Your belly will pick up the front of the dress or skirt. Maternity clothing is cut to hang a few inches longer in front to take up the belly.

- You will never use the oversized clothing after the baby is born, because it will be too large for you and your vanity will not permit you to wear it.

It is also unwise to make do with your own clothing or with someone else's maternity clothes unless they have terrific things. You will look sloppy and in the end will convey just the impression that you are trying to erase.

With this in mind, here are a few suggestions on how to make the most of your clothing needs:

Plotting Your Wardrobe

Don't rush into maternity clothing. Most women begin feeling the strain on their regular clothes at about three months. Think ahead and determine what, if any, plans you have for which you will need a specific type of clothing. For instance, if you know that during your seventh month you will be attending a formal wedding, then plan for that purchase when plotting your maternity wardrobe. If you know that you will be making an overseas trip, then consider your needs for that.

Consider the type of schedule you normally lead, and list the type of clothing you would probably purchase to fill the needs for these activities.

Myrna Tarnower, owner of Mater's Market, a New York City maternity boutique, suggests that you not buy everything at once, because if you stagger your purchasing you will give yourself a lift as your belly expands.

Tarnower, who is a nationally known designer and manufacturer of maternity wear, suggested the following purchasing program: In the third month, you should get one to two maternity dresses, one to two tops and/or sweaters, and maternity jeans and/or pants. You will then be prepared for the morning when you discover that you are unable to fit into your regular clothing.

Sometime during the fourth or fifth month, your waist begins to go. At this time you should purchase the basic core of your wardrobe. In the sixth month, you can purchase fill-in articles. During the eighth month, buy one article to give yourself a lift, because now begins the real expansion. In the ninth month, go out and buy yourself something for the hospital and something smashing for when you come home from the hospital. Be sure you have a comfortable robe that buttons or zips up the front to take to the hospital with you.

Body Shapes

Although manufacturers say they cannot design for individual body shapes (they size their clothing "petite," "junior" and "misses"), in fact certain styles are more flattering on some women than others.

At a leading New York department store, for instance, the maternity buyer explains that "we try to see the maternity customer as a shape. Certain clothing is definitely more flattering to certain body shapes."

You might want to consider the following guidelines regarding body shapes when looking for your maternity clothing:

If you are a big woman or are carrying large

- The tent dress is the most flattering silhouette for you.

- Jumpers and dresses are preferable.

- Avoid belting the garment.

- Look for softer fabrics and solid colors. The larger the pattern or stiffer the fabric, the larger you will look. You can always wear a small print blouse under the jumper or dress for contrast.

If you are tall (over 5'6")

- You may have trouble finding pants that are long enough for you. Ask the buyer in your local store if she can order them from the manufacturer. Most manufacturers feel there is no market in maternity clothes for the woman 5'6" and above. We suspect a market would emerge if the consumer would ask for the product.

If you are small or carrying small, almost everything will look good on you, but keep in mind the following:

- Clothing that is belted will suit you well. Belt the item under the bustline.

- Watch the hemline. If the item needs to be shortened, do it to avoid looking dumpy.

- Avoid skirts and short tops—they will tend to make you look stubby. If you want to wear skirts, then look for a longer top or a tunic top, which will give you a longer look.

In any case, look for items that will "grow" with you. Some maternity clothing has belts or special internal seams that can be easily slit open to expand the garment as your pregnancy progresses.

Your Wardrobe Components

There is absolutely no reason to be an unsightly pregnant woman. Although many would agree with the secretary who said, "I never found pregnancy particularly attractive, so I felt less attractive myself," *do* try and make the best of your changing figure. One public relations assistant put it this way: "Even if you are pregnant, it is important that clothing reflect a certain stature. And you cannot do that by wearing boxy tops with puffed sleeves, Peter Pan collars and bows at the neck. That kind of dressing just doesn't make it any more."

With this in mind, here are two basic suggested wardrobes for the working and nonworking woman. Since much of the maternity clothing available today spans seasons you will probably be able to collect items that concentrate on the layered look, thus enabling you to get more wear out of your selections. In warmer climates, dressing tends to be more casual anyway, so look for the same lightweight fabrics you would wear if you were not pregnant.

Suggested Maternity Wardrobes

Working

The working woman, because of her work and leisure activities, may want to consider the following:

    Day dresses, possibly one with a jacket (2–3)
    Jumpers (2)
    Day-to-dinner dress (1)
    Dinner dresses (2)
    Pants, possibly including one pantsuit (2)
    Tops and/or sweaters (4)
    Jeans (1)
    Active sportswear outfits (tennis, swimming, running) (optional)
    Coat or cape (optional)

Nonworking

The nonworking woman, because of her more casual life, may want to consider the following:

    Pants, possibly including two pantsuits (3–4)

Jumpers (1–2)
Evening outfits, including one dinner dress (1–2)
Tops and/or sweaters (4–5)
Jeans (1–2)
Shorts (1)
Active sportswear outfits (tennis, swimming, running) (optional)
Coat or cape (optional)

Accessories

Although you may not have considered wardrobe to mean anything other than clothing, there are a few other things to consider:

- *Shoes.* Wear comfortable shoes. High heels may cause back strain; flat shoes may cause varicose veins and leg cramps. Stick with a comfortable shoe that has a medium heel. You may also discover that your feet will tend to swell a bit more easily during pregnancy, so you may want to invest in one pair of shoes slightly larger than the size you normally wear.

- *Other accessories.* If you wear jewelry at all, keep it simple. Your necklaces may prove to be a bit tight around the neck and your hands may swell, making it difficult to remove your rings. If this happens, take the rings off and keep them off until after the delivery. If you are wearing belts, make sure they are small ones. Avoid large buckles because they may be uncomfortable resting on your belly.

- *Underwear.* Maternity underwear is widely available, and this includes bras, girdles, slips, underpants and panty hose. If they are not available in a maternity department, check the lingerie department of your local store. If you are planning to nurse, you may want to purchase your nursing bras now to save a trip back after delivery.

Hair, Skin and Teeth

You probably already know that the hormonal changes during pregnancy affect your hair, your skin and your teeth. Sometimes you will look beautiful; other times, not so terrific at all. Even if you have never given much thought to your appearance before, make a little extra effort during pregnancy. Do it for yourself.

- *Hair*. Get a terrific haircut at the beginning of your pregnancy, during the middle and shortly before your due date. You won't have time to get one for many weeks after you deliver, because the new baby, your family and visitors will keep you busy—and you will be trying to regain your strength.

  Anyone who colors her hair today knows there are considerable questions regarding the safety of certain hair dyes. Government warnings and studies currently advise against the potential carcinogenic effects of some chemicals used in these dyes, and there are many unanswered questions regarding not only what you put on your hair, but what fumes you may inhale during the process. Voice your concerns to your hairdresser and your physician, and discuss any natural alternatives that may be more acceptable for you during your pregnancy.

- *Skin*. Though some people experience a change in skin during pregnancy, not everyone does. If your skin is oily, use a cleanser and astringent and occasional deep-cleansing mask to tighten your pores and keep them clean. If your skin is dry, use a cleansing toner with a lower alcohol content, and a moisturizer at night.

- *Makeup*. Take a little extra care with your makeup, even if you never have before. You want to look natural and let your skin breathe, but be careful to highlight your features in as nonartificial a way as possible. As a general guideline, use less, but apply it with more care.

  Splurge, if you can, for a facial once or twice during your pregnancy. It not only will feel terrific and do wonders for your face, but it will give you a needed lift around the ninth month.

- *Teeth*. See your dentist early during your pregnancy and again toward the end. The increased hormonal secretions do tend to affect your gums, and may cause an increase in periodontal (gum) disease. Tell your dentist you are pregnant so that he will *not* take X-rays but will know to pay special attention to your gums.

One final word regarding the postpregnancy period. After you deliver you will be surprised to learn that no matter how many exercises you do, or how terrific a shape you are in, your belly will not be flat again for some time. You may think that you will be able to get into your clothing again right away, but you won't.

You certainly will not want to look at the maternity outfits that you have been wearing for months, no matter how terrific they were, yet your vanity will not let you believe that you are unable to get into your former clothing.

Be prepared for it. It may take days, weeks or months, but your belly will not return to its original shape the minute you recover from childbirth. This is especially true if you have a cesarean section, which is considered major abdominal surgery and usually results in swollen abdominal tissues and sore muscles.

So here's a hint. Save one dress for this transition period, or buy a special dress for this time. It will be something new, and you will look forward to wearing it.

You don't have to feel badly about not fitting into your clothing. This is something that happens to everyone, but no one talks about it. One famous stage star wore a set of transition maternity clothing for six months after the birth of her child. Everyone assumed it was part of her new postpregnancy look, which it was. She just never told anyone that it was mostly transition maternity clothing, and because she was no longer pregnant no one had the faintest idea of what she had done.

If you refuse to believe this will happen to you, ask the salesperson at the store where you purchased some of your clothing to hold a dress for you. Explain what you want it for and pay for it. Most will allow a short return period if you leave the tags on and do not wear the article. See what happens after childbirth—then make your decision. You may be very happy you have that dress.

THE NEW PREGNANCY

8

SEX AND SEXUALITY

There are new aspects of sexuality for you to explore during your pregnancy that can add a special dimension to it, bringing exceptional pleasure. Your belly proclaims you as a sexual being, and despite the many changes of pregnancy, your body and spirit are well able to respond— if you are free and willing.

"Pregnancy can be a marvelous sexual time," says Dr. Virginia Sadock, a Manhattan psychiatrist and sex therapist. "It's a physical demonstration of a woman's femaleness." When a happy sexual fillip is added to pregnancy, it is, says Dr. Lonnie Garfield Barbach of the University of California, "an incredibly positive thing. It is a way of saying, 'Not only do I love you, I love this baby and this process.' "

Pregnancy itself adds a certain sensuality, even by enlarging your breasts; the act of giving birth can raise you to a new degree of physical experience. Many women discover unsuspected joy in the warm exchange between their bodies and their newborns during cuddling or breast-feeding. Some men are particularly aroused by pregnancy; some women feel new levels of desire.

With all of this potential for pleasure and fulfillment, too many women and their partners have less than optimal sex lives during pregnancy. Sex is the start of pregnancy—pregnancy shouldn't mean the end of sex! Some women, some couples, have marvelous intimacy during pregnancy; others are less fortunate. Why should this happen? What about you?

To answer such questions, we have identified five major obstacles, any one of which may block your ability to be sexually alive during pregnancy. These obstacles are (1) the fear that sex will harm your baby; (2) the traditional prejudice against sexuality during pregnancy; (3) the common failure of the medical world to help women recognize the importance and nature of their sexuality during pregnancy, a failure compounded by erratic advice about sex during pregnancy; (4) the highly individual, ever-changing pattern of sexual response and desire in pregnancy and after childbirth that may baffle, surprise or dismay you; (5) the fact that for pregnancy the very definition of sexuality has to be expanded.

Pregnancy makes so many demands on your psyche, intelligence, body and energy, you may think that sex is just too much—or too unimportant—to concern you now. If so, you are wrong, because staying alive sexually can improve your pregnancy. "There is no time in a woman's life when she is as vulnerable and dependent and needs emotional support," says Dr. Sadock. "She needs support for her own identity, and nothing is more reassuring than to know that she is wanted."

To help you recognize and realize the sexual potential of your pregnancy, we first have to deal with some common obstacles.

OBSTACLE 1: FEAR AND HOW TO DISSOLVE IT

Without question, the most rocklike obstacle in the way of your sexual freedom during pregnancy is fear—your fear, or your partner's fear, that you will harm your unborn child. Luckily, with few exceptions and only slight modifications, *in general sex during pregnancy is considered safe.* Unluckily, not enough pregnant women and their partners know all the facts. Even if they do, fear can sometimes be so strong that a couple may avoid physical contact and sexual release.

Dr. Celia J. Falicov of the Community Psychology Program in Chicago did an in-depth study of the sexual adjustment of women in their first pregnancies. She found "a fear—frequently recognized as unrealistic—of harming the fetus or provoking a miscarriage interfered with readiness to engage in sexual intercourse for ten of nineteen . . . by the eighth month of pregnancy, fifteen of eighteen women had stopped sexual intercourse . . . it is interesting to note that in only five cases had the obstetrician advised the women to stop coital activity six to seven weeks prior to the delivery date. The other ten had read or heard that sexual abstinence was strongly recommended at this time."

Since you and your partner may be genuinely worried about the safety of sex during pregnancy, it is worth exploring the subject in some detail. As in every aspect of childbearing, new studies and headlines appear which may cause concern. In 1979, work was reported from the Hershey Medical Center in Pennsylvania which showed an increased risk of amniotic fluid infection, and therefore some infant deaths, when pregnant women had had sexual relations late in pregnancy, and more particularly, before a premature birth. Even at the time of the report in *The New England Journal of Medicine*, there was no attempt to advise all pregnant women from refraining from intercourse. By a year later, in December of 1980, an official of ACOG said in an interview that there had been no change in the general advice of "sex as long as it is enjoyable and comfortable" depending on a woman's individual health condition and obstetrical history.

What Science Says about Sex during Pregnancy

It is indicative of the value that medical science has placed on human sexuality in general and female sexuality in particular that although hundreds of scientific papers are published each year on obstetrics, the major studies about sex and pregnancy can be kept in a few manila folders. Some areas of controversy are unresolved, but enough is known to give you some answers to major questions.

Since the 1960's there has been a liberalizing shift in what obstetricians are taught. Where once there was a three-month ban on intercourse—from six weeks before delivery to six weeks after—obstetrical residents today learn that sexual activity can safely continue throughout healthy pregnancy. Whether or not it can safely continue in very late pregnancy is still a question looking for a definitive answer. The general attitude of the informed practicing obstetrician may be expressed by Dr. John D'Urso, a Manhattan obstetrician-gynecologist who delivers two hundred babies a year: "I tell my patients that unless there are problems, sex is absolutely normal throughout pregnancy. After the middle of the ninth month I ask them to be a little less aggressive because the cervical and vaginal tissues get softer."

If you are having a healthy pregnancy, you should expect your physician to tell you something similar. If he or she doesn't, you should ask why not.

Although medical texts (and probably most male physicians) speak of "coital activity" or "marital relations" in sex and pregnancy, when you ask about your safety you are really also asking about the effect of your experiencing an orgasm, which can occur quite independently of intercourse. Therefore, when you ask about sex—or you are given instructions—ask if your doctor is referring to intercourse or orgasm. It is during orgasm that several muscles, including that important protective muscle, your uterus, contracts.

Some studies have questioned whether or not the contractions of orgasm might cause fetal distress. Studying late pregnancy, when the spasms of contractions can naturally follow orgasm, researchers William Masters and Virginia Johnson have observed that "listening to the fetal heart tones at this time may return evidence of a slowed heart rate, but this reaction is transitory in character. No further evidence of fetal distress has been demonstrated."

One as yet unresolved question about sex during pregnancy is—can sex cause labor?

In the early 1950's Drs. William E. Pugh and Frank L. Fernandez of the Department of Obstetrics and Gynecology at the University of Louisville School of Medicine in Kentucky did a classic study on the effects of intercourse in late pregnancy, delivery and the postpartum period. More than five hundred patients in a hospital obstetric service were studied and watched for complications, such as premature rupture of the membranes, premature labor and bleeding. Pugh and Fernandez emphatically concluded that "coitus is not responsible for the various complications of late pregnancy, delivery, and the puerperium frequently attributed to it." This study is the basis for much of what obstetricians are taught about sex in late pregnancy.

Still there are questions. In the 1930's, hormones called prostaglandins, commonly found in semen, were discovered. It was learned that when prostaglandins are put on strips of uterine muscle in the laboratory, the muscle contracts. Whether or not prostaglandins are present in enough quantity in an ejaculation to cause labor isn't known. Women produce prostaglandins in small quantities, as well as oxytocin, which can be used by physicians in synthetic form to induce labor. One female obstetrician advises her pregnant patients who are overdue to have intercourse with a great deal of zeal—advice that is more enticing than the old wives' advice to scrub floors to bring on labor! Some cultures allow intercourse near term to help bring on delivery.

All of this is interesting, but it is not conclusive. In one study, five women at term were asked to have an orgasm at a scheduled time to see if they could induce labor. Four were able to orgasm for the sake of science; two went into labor within three hours; one within nine hours, and the fourth went into false labor. All had normal, healthy babies, uneventful deliveries and hospital stays. This is also not conclusive.

Since there are no definite answers, it is useful to consider informed opinion. In this case the opinion was written in a medical publication by Dr. Fritz Fuchs, professor of reproductive biology at the Cornell–New York Medical Center and coauthor of a major work that collates studies done in many nations on the hormones related to pregnancy. "It is my personal opinion," writes Dr. Fuchs, "that coitus may trigger labor if the uterus is very labile, but under normal circumstances it does not. In spite of the advice of the obstetrician to abstain from intercourse during the last six weeks of pregnancy, many patients prefer to please a husband rather than keep their obstetrician happy, and if coitus were likely to induce labor the incidence of premature labor would be much higher than it is."

Sex during Uncomplicated Pregnancy

It is a sign of loving concern on the parts of prospective mothers and fathers to worry about harming a baby, but the fetus is so well protected within its mother's body that the chance of actual direct physical trauma is slight.

You should know, however, that if there is any bleeding after intercourse, sex should be stopped and a visit to a physician scheduled. If sex is *ever* uncomfortable or painful for you, the activity should be stopped, the truth told and perhaps another position or activity tried. Toward the end of pregnancy, when the cervix is softening preparatory to opening during labor, penile thrusting can be uncomfortable. Intercourse is possible as long as it is not too violent.

In late pregnancy, if the membrane of the amniotic sac ruptures—detectable because there is a rush of fluid—sex should be avoided and a physician called right away.

Here are some specifics that may answer questions about sex practices and activities during pregnancy.

Positions. It has been estimated that there are some 600 different positions that have been devised for lovemaking. Therefore, if any particular position is uncomfortable for you during pregnancy, there are plenty of others. Many women and their partners worry that the traditional man-on-top (missionary) position may mean too much pressure on a pregnant belly. This is a particular concern in late pregnancy. While not harmful, this position may be less than enjoyable for you. Many couples use the woman-on-top position of intercourse. Another position to consider might be to have you lie on your side with your mate at your back, entering the vagina from behind you. A side-to-side position facing each other also might work well. During your pregnancy, there may be times when deep penetration is uncomfortable for you. You and your partner are aware of which positions promote penetration deep into the vagina to the cervix. You might want to choose or explore other positions that allow shallow penetration.

Sex Practices. Pregnancy does not mean a halt of sexual activities that you enjoy. For example, masturbation is fine, provided that there is no medical reason why you should avoid orgasm. As for vibrators, a number of experts were asked to comment on their use in the genital areas of pregnant women. None felt competent to make a statement. They noted, however, that a vibrator can provoke intense orgasms, which may stimulate uncomfortable uterine contractions. In late pregnancy there is the unanswered question—do intense contractions lead to labor? Given the unknowns, vibrators may not be a great idea during pregnancy.

As for oral sex, this is an activity that can be freely enjoyed. However, there is one form of oral sex that is very dangerous. It is called vaginal insufflation. In vaginal insufflation, air is forcefully blown into the vagina to create an impression of fullness. This practice is dangerous because it can cause life-threatening air embolisms.

Another sexual practice, a switching back and forth between vaginal and anal penetration, calls for a precaution during pregnancy. The anus is a reservoir for the microscopic life forms that cause vaginal infections. Hence, if this sexual practice is one that you favor, your partner should wash or wear a condom before reentering your vagina. Pregnancy already makes you prone to vaginal infection, and there is no reason to increase your susceptibility through a sexual practice. You needn't abandon the practice, just modify it.

Another precaution: Hot tubs and saunas—which some women use as a pleasing and sensual experience—may not be advisable during pregnancy. Some reports have linked high temperatures to an increased risk of birth defects.

Sex and High-Risk Pregnancy

There are some medical situations that call for prohibitions on sexual activity. You should, of course, heed your physician's advice. But some traditional strictness about sex in troubled pregnancy has been eased. For example, miscarriage is very common in early pregnancy. Traditionally, women with a history of prior miscarriage have been told to refrain from sex. Though every woman needs individualized medical advice on this matter, this flat sex restriction no longer holds true. Medical science now has the capacity to diagnose the cause of many miscarriages. If, for example, the loss of a fetus was attributed to the fact that the fetus was defective—a very common reason for miscarriage—there may be no valid reason to prohibit sex in later pregnancies. Dr. John W. Grover, assistant clinical professor of obstetrics and gynecology at the Harvard Medical School, said in an article directed at physicians: "Because of their predictably high levels of anxiety and emotional tension, couples with prior multiple miscarriages or midtrimester losses need careful and individual attention during a present pregnancy. When no discernible cause is apparent, couples may continue their loving and satisfying sexual relationship without fear of harm to the pregnancy . . . One should differentiate those conditions in which orgasm is contraindicated from those in which vaginal penetration is hazardous. It is extremely helpful in these difficult situations to involve both partners in the management and progress of the pregnancy."

If, for any reason, you are told to abstain from sex during pregnancy, ask what is specifically being prohibited. If intercourse alone is being prohibited, there are other pleasurable ways to achieve orgasm. There may be favorite alternatives that both you and your partner enjoy. If you want to try something new, there are many books about sexual methods that are written in a way to inform, not shock. Begin with an alternative sexual activity that is the least bizarre and threatening to you and your partner. You may find new horizons in sexuality as a bonus of your pregnancy if you treat a medical "no sex" as a challenge instead of as a prohibition.

If you are to avoid orgasm, you have to be realistic and understand that you are only going to be miserable or resentful if you are partially stimulated but allowed no real release. This doesn't mean that you should deny yourself the joy of intimacy, but it does mean that you should exclude unfair stimulation. You can ask your partner to bypass touching your breasts or genitals and give you a neck massage or tummy rub if this is a pleasant but not especially erotic experience for you. If "no orgasm" means that you must stop self-stimulation, you should try to treat yourself to some sensual experience rather than feel totally deprived. This could mean splurging on a gift for yourself or a treat that you will really enjoy.

OBSTACLE 2: PREJUDICE AND HOW TO BYPASS IT

Your sexuality is one subject that the world would like to forget, but it is too important for too many fine reasons for *you* to forget. The prejudice against sexuality during pregnancy can take many forms. It may be expressed in the words or actions of your sexual partner or of strangers on the street, or in your own feelings about how you look naked and how you rate your own sexual desirability. It may even influence your readiness to participate in sexual activity during pregnancy. Dr. Lonnie Garfield Barbach says, "During pregnancy a lot of women look better than they ever have in their lives. Pregnancy makes them self-assured, and *that* turns men on. Everything about sex is so idiosyncratic. Some men prefer women who are overweight. They like certain body types."

Said a willowy fashion model with an eight-month belly, "I have no shyness about my body, and I love being pregnant. I get a lot of reinforcement by having people admire me. I think that it would be terrible to go through pregnancy without having someone tell you that you look great." And if no one tells you that you look great—tell it to yourself.

To many women the ultimate test of attractiveness is to be desired. We can think of no more vivid proof to offer you that a pregnant woman *is* sexually desirable than to share this true story:

In her third pregnancy, a Michigan woman had her first love affair outside of marriage. She didn't expect it or plan it. It happened in her first trimester, when women are supposed to have the least sexual desire or interest. It happened when she was thirty-five, when women are supposed to be finished as sexual prizes. It happened with a man she had known for years. "I was hypersexual, and my husband just wasn't going through these incredible feelings and changes. I needed someone who responded to me in the same positive sensual way I was feeling. The man who became my lover had no hang-ups or taboos."

While no one is advocating affairs during pregnancy, it is nice to know that they can happen—particularly since they usually work the other way round!

Vaginal Discharge

Every woman, pregnant or nonpregnant, has some form of vaginal discharge. In pregnancy, vaginal discharge increases because of mucus secreted by the cervix and other influences, such as sexual stimulation. Pregnancy also makes you more vulnerable to the development of vaginal infection because of changes in your physiological balance. These infections can cause a variety of unpleasant symptoms, including itching, swollen tissues, painful intercourse, and occasionally an unpleasant-smelling discharge.

No woman is happy about vaginal discharge, but don't punish yourself by being embarrassed about a normal event. Your physician can advise you about treatment for vaginal infection, if it is required. Discuss treatment pros and cons, because the vagina absorbs drugs quickly. Also, if ever you had genital herpes, a viral genital infection, before your pregnancy, be sure to alert your physician because a recurrence during pregnancy can be a problem.

Good hygiene can do a lot to help you prevent an outbreak of symptoms from a vaginal infection. This includes washing the vulva area each day with a mild soap; using only your personal washcloth and towel; changing your underwear; avoiding nylon underthings or panty hose, choosing instead cotton lingerie or cotton-lined underthings. Douching is not recommended during pregnancy.

The use of perfumed sprays, the so-called feminine hygiene products, is out because these irritants can initiate vaginal problems. We use these products because we have been trained to think of our intimate parts and functions as unclean. We are perfectly fine as we are, but if you or your partner prefer another scent, an aromatic oil rubbed on your belly or along your hips can be erotic without harming you.

What Is Your Mate Thinking?

Sexuality is obviously equally important to your mate. Men are not free of mixed reactions to sex and pregnancy. One lawyer, whose wife is pregnant with their first child, says, "I have to admit that I had had some hang-ups about sex and pregnancy. My mother got pregnant when I was fourteen years old, and I was embarrassed even to be near her. It was an admission that she had a sex life at forty-four, and that bothered me."

In *Making Love During Pregnancy,* a beautifully illustrated volume about the sexual experiences of couples who had taken prepared childbirth classes, Elizabeth Bing and psychologist Libby Colman noted, "The husband may wish that his wife's body would stay as it was. Her new superfeminine body, her heavier scent, her extra lubrication, and her increased engorgement may be frightening, almost overwhelming." They observed that this reaction may cause a man to lose an erection, and that changes in a couple's patterns and practices of sex may seem "regressive and unclean."

Many men have very positive reactions to the sexuality of pregnancy. A thirty-year-old Texas store owner said, "My wife walked and acted throughout her pregnancy as if pregnancy was the highest state of being. She always had extremely nice breasts, but when she was pregnant they were even nicer. She was a fascination to me. For me, her pregnancy was a sexual high."

Some men may have negative reactions, and this should be worked out by talking. The most dangerous sexual practice during pregnancy is not sexual at all—it is a lack of communication about what is happening in your sex lives and your feelings about each other. As we will see when we discuss the changing patterns of sexuality during pregnancy, there can be shifts in desire and a few body changes that may influence sexual response. If you and your mate anticipate that changes might occur, you will be able to deal with them if they do. Some researchers have noted that men don't know about the sexual aspects of pregnancy. Unless your mate has access to childbirth education classes or feels comfortable speaking with a physician, it really is up to you to pass along the facts about sex during pregnancy. Where do you get your facts and advice? That's the next obstacle to tackle.

OBSTACLE 3: ERRATIC ADVICE ON EROTIC MATTERS, OR HOW TO DEAL WITH A FLAW IN THE MEDICAL PROFESSION

Pregnant women who speak together quickly learn that what one is told about sex—or is not told—depends on her choice of doctor. By cleverly picking a physician known to be liberal, a healthy woman may be "permitted" to have sexual intercourse throughout pregnancy. Another doctor in the same community may automatically say "no sex" beginning four or even six weeks before the due date.

Women can talk to other women, read, or turn to their obstetricians or medical team for information, guidance, advice, help about sexual relations and feelings during pregnancy. ACOG maintains that it is one of the four prime functions of a specialist to be a sex guidance counselor. Not all obstetricians deserve the title.

Many women we interviewed said they felt that they could discuss anything with their obstetricians. Other women tried but were unsuccessful.

A high school teacher we spoke to who has been pregnant twice and had changed her obstetrician-gynecologist largely because of his failure to help her with sexual problems related to pregnancy felt that "most doctors, especially older ones, are unable to deal with any kind of sexuality issues or discuss sexual feelings from a woman's point of view. Even when they ask the right questions, they don't really want to stop and hear the answers." She was in an anxious state during her first pregnancy about her "overwhelming and unusual desire for sex," and she was worried because she and her husband were having problems with their sex life. It was doubly difficult for her to talk to her obstetrician with dignity and confidence, because she was dressed in a paper robe that barely covered her belly.

Almost a year after the birth of her first child, this woman returned for a routine gynecological checkup. She told her doctor that she and her husband had a totally unsatisfactory sex life, and that they were miserable. She asked him to recommend someone—a psychiatrist or sex therapist, a professional—who could help. He absolutely ignored that request, and suggested that she and her husband go to a motel. She later discovered that this was his standard suggestion for any sexual question raised by a patient. She then went to her internist, who told her to go home and stop worrying. Here are two men in positions of authority who didn't help at all.

The attitude and prejudices of an obstetrician-gynecologist can be very strong. When medical authority is added to that, what pregnant women can be told about sex can be overwhelming—and wrong!

Why Your Physician May Be Less than a Help about Sexual Matters

Physicians are trained and adept at many different requirements of their profession, but only very, very recently has human sexuality been a subject of study and concern. Even today, although many medical schools include sex education in their curriculum, not all do. Sexuality is just not a high medical priority, however important it is to people. ACOG has only recently prepared special educational materials and offered continuing education courses in human sexuality. As for obstetrics, although the importance of a patient's sex life during pregnancy is beginning to get some attention, many obstetricians have little time or inclination to be of real help to patients with questions. *Williams Obstetrics,* the most respected medical textbook on obstetrics in this country, for example, devotes just a few paragraphs to sexuality. Also, there can be a lag between research findings related to sexuality and a change in the attitudes of physicians and what they tell their patients.

"There can be a failure among gynecologists to keep up with the latest advances," said Dr. Harold Lief, professor of psychiatry and director of the Division of Family Study at the University of Pennsylvania School of Medicine.

"But the work of Masters and Johnson and work on the safety of sex has been known since the 1960's."

If you encounter a negative attitude on the part of a physician, an unwillingness to discuss sexual matters, or even indifference, don't be surprised. There has been a long history of negative, distorted and often very prejudiced medical attitudes towards female sexuality. Despite this generally unhelpful medical attitude, it is important for you to at least try to speak with your physician.

Getting Answers from the Medical World

It is a chore at times to broach the subject of sexuality with an obstetrician—particularly during a rushed office visit. Nonetheless, it is important to do so and to be as specific as you can. If you find your physician reacting poorly to your questions or your need to talk about sexuality, or if you find him condemning any practice without a good medical reason, you might consider changing doctors. If you have a real sexual problem and you are not being helped by your obstetrician, you might consider sex therapy. In general, sex therapists say that pregnancy is not the time to go into sex therapy unless there is a real need, because there are so many emotions and life and body changes taking place all at once. Besides, your problem may not be that unusual or lasting.

Don't be surprised if you experience sexual feelings towards your obstetrician or have fantasies. Some women do because of the power mystique of physicians or because their obstetricians know intimate details about them and accept the fact that they are pregnant.

Whatever your attitude, since your physician is a major source of information about sexuality and knows your pregnancy, you should try to at least work at communication.

OBSTACLE 4: CONFUSING ASPECTS OF SEXUALITY DURING PREGNANCY, OR WHAT'S HAPPENING?

Pregnancy is an overwhelming experience that can throw your emotions into disorder and create chaos in your relationships. One moment you may find yourself without desire, the next moment erotically supercharged. Pregnancy is nine long months, and the lack of interest you may feel in your first nauseated trimester may turn into passion a month later. Many pregnant women and their partners are just not prepared for change in their pattern or tempo of intimacy, so we'll help explain what's going on in your body.

What Happens to Your Pregnant Body during Sex

Two outstanding sex researchers of recent years—Masters and Johnson—have done important research that established objective proof of the sexual capability of pregnant women. Our growing bodies do become excited and respond. While every woman's identification and definition of orgasm is personally correct for her, it is useful to understand what happens in scientifically observed sexual response during pregnancy.

Through their major research, Masters and Johnson have established a normal four-phase female sexual response cycle. It begins with sexual "excitement" or arousal, moves into a "plateau" stage, which prepares the way for the "orgasm" stage, which is followed by "resolution," when the body returns to its normal resting state. This cycle is for women, pregnant and nonpregnant.

In addition to studying the sexual response cycle of nonpregnant women, Masters and Johnson also did laboratory studies of the same response cycle in pregnant women. Here is what normally happens in the response cycle—phase by phase—and what happens in each phase during pregnancy:

Nonpregnancy Phase One—The "Excitement" Phase

A woman is sexually aroused by whatever works that magic for her, be it mate, an erotic thought, self-stimulation or a vibrator. Blood rushes to swell her sexual organs, including her sensitive clitoris. She may become lubricated. Her vagina, a hollow tube of elastic muscle, expands and

becomes longer; her uterus shifts slightly to make room
for a penis; her breasts may swell and her nipples may
become erect.

Pregnancy Phase One—The "Excitement" Phase

When a pregnant woman becomes sexually aroused, it is
important to remember that pregnancy has already caused
her pelvis and genitals to have a richer blood supply.
Through the first two trimesters, when arousal occurs the
minor outer lips become very much engorged with blood;
by the third trimester, this whole area is so swollen by
pregnancy that the added swelling of sexual organs because of excitement is difficult to detect in a laboratory.
Whereas a nonpregnant women may become lubricated
during excitement, the pregnant woman may already have
increased lubrication.

In the first trimester, as the fetus grows and the uterus
moves up into the abdomen, the vagina continues to
extend and lengthen during the excitement phase, as it
does in nonpregnant women. However, after the uterus
elevates, part of the vaginal wall "tents" to an extent that
it is not possible to measure its direct response to sexual
stimulation.

Breast response is often part of the normal excitement
phase. And in pregnancy, when enlarged breasts can
account for as much as one and a half pounds of total
weight gain, a rush of blood because of sexual excitement
can cause tenderness and pain, particularly in the first
trimester and especially for women in their first pregnancy. This fades later in pregnancy.

Nonpregnancy Phase Two—The "Plateau" Phase

A women's entire genital area, the outer lips and part of
the vagina, swell even more with an onrush of blood. The
opening of the vagina constricts and forms what is called
the "orgasmic platform," which contains and can tighten
around a penis or object. Muscles elsewhere in the body—
as close to the genital action as pelvic and thigh muscles,

as distant as facial muscles—tense. The moment of orgasm approaches.

Pregnancy Phase Two—The "Plateau" Phase

In the pregnant women Masters and Johnson studied, whether or not it was a first pregnancy, sexual tension created huge engorgement of the "orgasmic platform" and a swelling of vaginal walls to the extent that instead of being the curved walls of a hollow tube, the sides of the vagina touch. This laboratory finding explains why many women—and their men—report that "there is no room" or the vagina is "too tight."

Nonpregnancy Phase Three—"Orgasm"

Although every woman has her own definition of what orgasm is and feels like, in the laboratory orgasm is recorded in terms of contractions of the orgasmic platform, the muscles of the uterus and, perhaps, the anal sphincter muscles. Orgasm releases the blood that sexual tension sent cascading to target sexual organs—the clitoris, vagina and breasts—and so begins the final phase of female sexual response.

Pregnancy Phase Three—"Orgasm"

In the pregnant women they studied, Masters and Johnson were able to record orgasmic platform contractions during the first two trimesters. In the third trimester, although women can report contractions of the platform, the outer third of the vagina may be so engorged with blood and the entire vagina so swollen because of pregnancy that "Objective evidence of contractile efficiency is reduced markedly." Masters and Johnson also reported that in the last few weeks of pregnancy, instead of normal orgasmic contractions, the uterus may go into a form of spasm. By the end of pregnancy, following orgasm, a woman's supersensitive uterus may continue to contract for a while irregularly and her womb may feel like a hard mass of tightened muscle. This is a response that can be expected and is not a cause of worry. But you should always discuss it with your doctor.

Nonpregnancy Phase Four—"Resolution"

Essentially, this is a time of muscle relaxation, when the agitated swelled tissues and muscles go back to their presexual excitement state.

Pregnancy Phase Four—"Resolution"

It is in this phase that a pregnant woman's bodily responses differ. It takes far longer for the blood rushed to sexual target organs to return to the rest of the body, and as pregnancy advances, the blood concentration in the pelvis may not be relieved. For this reason, a woman in her second or third trimester may find herself feeling sexual tension or very sexually stimulated. It also may explain why some women do not feel relieved or released after a sexual experience.

Shifting Levels of Desire and Activity

Nothing about sexuality during pregnancy can be labeled normal for all women. As Dr. Lonnie Garfield Barbach of the Human Sexuality Program of the University of California Medical Center, author of *For Yourself; The Fulfillment of Female Sexuality,* said in an interview, "It's valuable to let women know that whether they feel turned on sexually during pregnancy or turned off; whether they feel like masturbating; whether they want an orgasm; whether they can or can't get a release—their feelings are all right and normal. They are the unique responses of each woman to the emotional and physiological changes which occur during pregnancy."

There can be fluctuations in desire or sexual contact—and these fluctuations can happen at any time during pregnancy or the postpartum period.

Some studies have been done of patterns of sexual behavior during pregnancy, documenting the kinds of fluctuations that we have mentioned. In general, women experienced reduced sexuality in the first trimester, an increase in the second trimester, and a decline in the third trimester, but there *are* variations.

"Women with high ratings on sexuality were less ambivalent or conflicted about sexual relations during pregnancy, and experienced fewer and milder changes and more sexual enjoyment than women who obtained low ratings," wrote Dr. Celia Falicov, who did a detailed study of pregnant women.

Remember: (1) Fluctuations can occur—so be aware. (2) Even when drops in sexual activity occur in groups of women, some women do better. Therefore, you should ask yourself, Is my reaction a lack of desire or a reflection of taboo? (3) You may be surprised by intense feelings of sexuality during your pregnancy. (4) Don't jump to negative conclusions about you and your sex life.

What Happens after Childbirth?

It's not fair—or wise—to look at the subject of sex and pregnancy without looking ahead to what can happen sexually after childbirth. Is it an automatic case of "and then they lived happily ever after"? Are women "ruined" by childbirth? Is the vaginal area "too loose" to allow pleasure? Does motherhood dim sexual desire?

In this country women are traditionally advised to avoid intercourse until their postpartum checkup, which can be from four to six weeks after delivery. Technically, a woman (who should remember that birth control is once again necessary) could have intercourse within two or three weeks after birth, once postpartum bleeding has stopped and any vaginal tear or episiotomy repair has healed. "Although the female may be physiologically capable of resuming coition early in the postpartum period, she may or may not be psychologically ready to do so," noted Masters and Johnson.

In terms of sexuality, the postpartum period can be what psychiatrist and sex therapist Virginia Sadock calls "a very sensitive time psychologically. The physical aspect of childbirth may have been either gratifying or traumatic, and then there is the reality factor—nothing interferes more with sex life than lack of sleep, and, of course, that's common with a new baby. The nurturance of the mother is being taxed. There is the whole reality of assuming parental identity. New parents need to give themselves a little breathing space. They have lost some of their privacy. If they can financially afford to do it, a weekend away together could be incredible."

Dr. Falicov noted that even seven months after childbirth, ten of the nineteen couples she studied were having intercourse less frequently than before pregnancy. She commented, "This seemed to be primarily the result of fatigue and sexual tension, since sexual desire and eroticism had returned to normal or heightened levels."

And that is an interesting paradox, one to keep in mind in what can be a slow readjustment period for some new parents. Whether it's the increased blood supply of pregnancy or her new attitude, a woman who has borne a child may have an increased orgasmic capacity.

Women—particularly those who have done pelvic and vaginal muscle exercises as part of childbirth preparation—have no reason to lose anything in terms of vaginal ability, because the vagina is a muscle designed for stretching. After birth, if there is any pain or discomfort during sex, the matter should be discussed with a gynecologist because there may be a physical problem that can be corrected.

Some women are displeased with the way they look after giving birth because of stretch marks, which will fade in time, but which will disappear only through cosmetic surgery. Some women who deliver by cesarean section are fortunate to have the incision made in the horizontal fold above the pubis, which makes the scar barely visible. Other women wind up with vertical scars that extend up from the pubis almost to the navel. Women do need a period to adjust to body scars, whether they are stretch marks or incisions. A man also has to have time to become used to a scar on the body of his lover.

OBSTACLE 5: THE NEED FOR A NEW DEFINITION OF SEX AND PREGNANCY

For the New Pregnancy that you are living, there has to be a new and better definition of sexuality, one that you must write for yourself. It will go beyond the fact or frequency of intercourse. There are many expressions of love. And remember, everything is normal.

You can grow as a sexual being if pregnancy helps you realize that not all of sex is intercourse or intercourse in one position or even orgasm.

"For a woman to have the physical warmth of closeness, to have her stomach rubbed, to have her husband give her a shampoo, these comforting things are important," says Dr. Sadock.

There is no denying that many demands are made of us in our lives, and pregnancy adds more strain. There also is no denying that relaxation and openness improve sex. Although it may be difficult, you have to find time for sex. It is no accident, for example, that therapeutic programs designed to help women achieve an orgasm insist that a woman set aside an hour each day to do sensuality training. This helps a woman learn about herself, and gives sexuality a true importance. Relax. And allow yourself time for enjoyment. You will discover many unexpected pleasures.

9

POSTPARTUM

The New Pregnancy does not end with childbirth.

As soon as your baby is born, you will discover that you are traveling on a new road, must quickly change gears and need a good set of directions fast. No amount of baby books or advice from others can prepare you for the practical realities of dealing with a newborn—or for the effect it will have on your life.

You may have had an active pregnancy, a wonderful health care and prepared childbirth experience, and a terrific relationship with your mate. You may have your plans for the future perfectly arranged, or be as confident as the couple who did not have one baby bottle in the house because they were sure that the mother would be able to breast-feed without any problems. (They discovered otherwise at three in the morning their first night home from the hospital.)

You will probably not be prepared, however, for the constant fatigue, for the complete dependency of a newborn or for your concerns about how well you are able to care for your baby the first few weeks after birth.

You will probably also be unprepared when those first guilt pangs of the motherhood mystique rear up to confront you and challenge your decision to return to work after a brief maternity leave; or for the guilt pangs that challenge your decision to stay home with your baby.

You may well be unprepared for the difficulties of

dealing with a spouse who suddenly discovers that the baby must inevitably come first, and that you are very tired at the end of a day even though you have "done nothing" but take care of a baby.

We are, therefore, going to try to give you a sense of this initial postpartum period—even though you may be certain that *none* of this will happen to you.

First, there is the question of how to handle the immediate postpartum period. This does *not* mean dealing with the emotional ups and downs you may experience after the baby is born. This means coping with an infant who is completely dependent upon you, and dealing with the physical and emotional fatigue that accompanies this dependency. Even if you have help, whether it be for the first few weeks after childbirth or longer, there will be times when you will be completely in charge and when you will be exhausted. Secondly, we will discuss dealing with the conflict that may arise when *your* perceptions about modern motherhood do not agree with the attitudes of those around you.

No woman should be punished for her pregnancy, nor should she have to apologize for it. No mother should have to feel guilty about wanting to care for her baby's needs and demands, nor should a woman be penalized for wanting to combine both a career and a family. And neither should she be criticized for her decision—whatever that may be.

For those women who opt for "Occupation: Outside Working Mother," this chapter will tell you how to deal with comments regarding your commitment to your baby, how to deal with guilt about your baby back home when you are at work, how to plan for backup help and contingencies, and how to reenter the work force with as few problems as possible.

For those women who opt for "Occupation: Inside Working Mother," this chapter will talk about the need to maintain your self-respect. We will discuss how to avoid feeling guilty about not working—when it appears that everyone around you is doing just that. In addition, we will discuss how other women have handled the common problems of isolation, lack of free time and loss of childless friends.

Finally, this chapter will talk about your relationship with your mate in the postpartum period. In this section, we will examine dual responsibilities and the development of a parenting scheme, whether you work or not.

THE PRACTICAL REALITIES OF DEALING WITH A NEWBORN

No matter how well prepared you are for pregnancy and childbirth, no one can really prepare you for the fatigue, both physical and emotional, that comes from the twenty-four-hour daily, weekend and holiday attention that a newborn requires. Every woman is different, and every family responds differently to the experience.

Those first few weeks after childbirth, however, are physically difficult and emotionally draining. Many women (as well as their spouses) feel anxious about coping and are overwhelmed by the responsibilities of caring for a newborn. In addition, many share common fears about the practical everyday duties associated with child care—simple things like feeding, diapering and burping. In order to help new families through this initial transition period, many more hospitals and childbirth education groups are now offering postpartum support groups to help parents deal with these common problems and anxieties.

"When you first bring the baby home," a thirty-two-year-old corporate whiz woman (who is well known in the New York business community for her managerial talents) said, "you are afraid that you are going to harm the baby. You don't know how to hold him, to feed him. You are afraid to put him down when he cries or pick him up when he doesn't. You are afraid something is wrong if he sleeps too long, or that something is wrong if he doesn't sleep enough. I was so sure that I was doing something wrong that every few hours I put a mirror under the baby's nose to make sure he was still breathing."

Just because you are a success at your job, on the tennis court or in the kitchen does not mean that these skills will automatically be transferred to successful infant care. You may well have a rough few weeks, so try and have realistic expectations about what the initial postpartum period will bring.

It is great when you are in the hospital and can press a button for service, or when your clean, fresh and dry baby is brought to you by a competent nurse who has to work only a seven- or eight-hour shift.

You will have left the hospital exhilarated with your baby, delighted to be the mother of a terrific little bundle, but once you reach your home you will be surprised at how quickly the situation gets out of hand and fatigue sets in. You will never be able to anticipate just how exhausting those first few weeks can be.

And even if you have heard how rough it is, you will probably underestimate it anyway—or think that *you* will handle it differently. Try to have realistic expectations about this initial transition. Remember, pregnancy and childbirth are times of stress and change. You must now learn to adjust to a new part of your life and to cope with these initial new anxieties.

Most women are complete novices at infant care. There is nothing to be ashamed of if you feel totally overwhelmed. Don't be afraid to admit your concerns.

The emotional responsibility of a newborn is awesome, even if you have help, and it is up to you to make the transition as smooth as possible.

In order to aid this transition, here are a few suggestions:

• *Keep telling yourself that you cannot do everything now— and then stick with it.* Try to avoid emotional overload, and concentrate on getting yourself and your family through those first few sleepless weeks. If you position your new group as a "family" rather than as a group of individuals (mother, father, baby), it will make your husband and any other children feel more like participants. They will be more willing to pitch in and and help if they think they are part of the action.

If you are planning to return to work, plan on not working at home those first few weeks. It is just one more thing to think about. You have taken on a major responsibility, so drop all other ones for the present. Don't spread yourself too thin.

Your body has gone through a terrific experience. Listen to it. Ask questions. Admit you are tired. And ask for help if you need it.

Overload brings fatigue, and the more tired you are the

more anxious you will be about your ability to cope with the demands of your baby. So get your rest, drop all excess responsibilities and concentrate on learning the many different aspects of child care.

- *Try to do a little preplanning.* Many women complain of the emotional responsibility more than any other aspect of the postpartum period. This often means that although you may have help, you are responsible for directing the help, or that although your husband may do the shopping, you have to tell him what to get. It means that you are mentally overloaded as far as continuously having to think and plan for those around you—and this can be as trying as the three o'clock in the morning feeding and a baby that does not want to go back to sleep.

  Try to plan a basic master list once a week with your help and spouse. Ask them to help you plan the requirements for the week in terms of errands, supplies, cleaning, and so on. Soon you will see some of the excess responsibility gradually drift over to the others.

- *Find someone to talk with to share your fears.* This may be someone in your prepared childbirth class, your prenatal class or postpartum support group. It may be a friend who recently had a baby.

  If you are lucky enough to have a nurse or other help, talk to her. Ask her to show you how to handle the baby. This is her job, and she probably knows it well or you would not have hired her. Don't be afraid to ask. Then listen and watch.

  If you are dissatisfied with your nurse or pediatrician, don't be afraid to change. The chemistry must be right.

  When you are reading the baby books, as every new mother does, keep in mind that they can only dispense general advice. Your baby may not conform to the generalities these books tend to speak in, so keep a flexible attitude and open mind and *use your common sense.* Oftentimes your best source for tips is other mothers who have recently gone through similar childbirth and infancy experiences.

- *Seriously consider whether you want your immediate family around the first few weeks.* Do you want them for a brief visit or as help? If your family does come to help, it will probably be your mother or mother-in-law. You might want to remember that her ideas about babies and children and yours may not be the same. And times have changed since she had her babies.

Think about the relationship you have with her and how she thinks about childrearing. If you are planning to return to work and your mother believes a woman belongs at home with her children, you may experience more conflict and tension than is necessary during this postpartum period.

Talk this out with your spouse—and when you extend the invitation to your family, make it explicit what type of visit and how long you expect it to be.

- *Try not to entertain the first few weeks.* Everyone will want to see the new baby, but try to stagger your visitors. And don't feel you have to serve an elaborate meal or snack to those who do come. Your childless friends may not completely understand what you are going through, so don't be upset if they expect you and your husband to be living the same way you were before the baby arrived.

- *Do not call your obstetrician unless you have medical questions about your own body.* An obstetrician is concerned with maternal health—not with the infant. It is natural for you to feel close to your obstetrician or health support team, but the questions about the baby should be directed toward your pediatrician. Many women suffer emotional setbacks when they discover that their obstetricians are not as interested in their welfare as they were prior to childbirth. Their major concern is *prenatal* development, and you have entered the postnatal period, so keep this in mind before making the phone call about your mother/child questions.

- *Let someone else do the wash and housecleaning.* Either hire someone, insist that your husband do it, or let it pile up until you regain your strength. If your help was not hired to do cleaning and wash (and most do not do it), do not expect it. If you press it, you may find yourself without help. You need to concentrate on building up your strength now to deal with the emotional needs of the baby, so let the housework slide for a while.

If you do not have the money to hire someone to give you a hand with the housework and your spouse balks about helping you, try to talk it out. Explain that you realize that he is tired when he comes home from work, but you are too. You might say that this is a transition time for you as a family, and you would appreciate his help in organizing your joint household responsibilities over the next month or two.

Then let him gradually organize himself into helping with the housework.

- *Get away by yourself at least a few minutes each day.* Sit down when the baby naps, and relax. Do nothing. You do not have to be a wonder woman now. You don't have to have dinner on the table when your husband comes home. It can wait—and he can help. The baby needs you first, and you need that time to catch a second wind.

- *Consider alternating the night feeding with your husband or helper the first few weeks.* Or you can handle the night feedings and let your male sleep so that he can take the morning feeding when he is up. That way you can sleep a little longer in the morning until the baby wakes for the next feeding.

- *Remember that it won't last forever.* The first few weeks are the worst, the next few weeks are better, and by the time the baby gets to be eighteen months old, your troubles will be over. By that time you will have forgotten how rough this initial period has been.

- *Try to get away for a day or two around the fifth or sixth week after childbirth.* If you can possibly swing a brief getaway, try to do it. Leave the baby at home with a nurse, family member or competent caretaker. The baby will do just fine without you for this brief period of time. You need this time to reestablish your relationship with your mate away from the daily pressures and demands of a small child.

  If you are unable to afford a few days or a weekend, then try to spend at least one night alone and away from the house with your husband. It will be a rejuvenating experience—you will rediscover your mate and return refreshed to begin your child-care duties again.

- *Keep your sense of humor.* There will be good days and bad days, happy days and irritable days. Keep your sense of humor and go with the flow.

POSTPARTUM CONFLICT

Whether you work or not, most likely your initial conflicts during this period will revolve around the care your baby is getting—either from you or from your help.

After you have passed the first few weeks, however, a

new set of concerns may emerge. If you are planning to return to work, you may experience a twinge of guilt regarding your decision. Many working women have said that their biggest fear may be discovering that they enjoy being at home with their baby.

Think about this. If you do enjoy the caretaking, consider whether you would want to do this all the time, talk it over with your spouse (and with your employer if you intend to return to work), and make your decision accordingly. There should be absolutely no stigma attached to the joy of being a full-time mother. And if you think you really would prefer to stay home and take care of your baby, then do it.

You may also decide that this may be a perfect time to consider a break in your work—or you may want to use this opportunity to consider a change in career plans. You should not have to feel guilty about not working, nor should you have to apologize for your baby.

Most working women are hit by two sets of conflicting needs during the postpartum period. If you plan to work, one concern is how much the baby is going to need you. The other is how much the office is going to miss you while you are away on maternity leave.

If you plan to stay home, you may feel conflicted about being there—and experience intensive emotional demands and isolation.

These conflicts are perfectly normal. On the one hand, you may feel that you should stay at home with the baby for the first few years; on the other hand, you may belong to the school that says that the quality of time devoted by a mother to a child is more important than the quantity.

Whatever your decision, you may be influenced by the attitudes of those around you. The most important thing for you to remember is that this is your decision. Do not make your decision by what others think you should do. Do what is best for you.

Being a Working Mother Entails Compromise

For those of you who are planning to return to work outside the home, you will require flexibility and the ability to set priorities and follow them. You will have to avoid overload and take a practical and unemotional ap-

proach to the many problems that will inevitably arise.
You must learn to function with as little guilt as possible.
In order to do this, decide what is important to you and
forget about the nonessentials. And doing both jobs, even
though you're tired, can be very gratifying. You'll have
the best of both worlds.

Fear of failure. The first attitude is the fear of failure
and is often caused by uncertainty about one's ability to
handle the many new responsibilities a baby entails plus
the routine work and domestic responsibilities carried
before. You may feel overwhelmed by your new dual
responsibilities, and fear that you won't be able to handle
everything. Truthfully, you probably won't, and this is as
good a time as any to begin thinking realistically about
the future relationship of your work and your family life.

Try and define what your concept of success is and,
conversely, what you fear you won't be able to accomplish because of your new dual roles. You *do* have a
major new responsibility, and even if you are not the one
caring for that baby all day, you are the one thinking
about it—and that is a very heavy responsibility in itself.

The mother who returns to a job outside the home may
find that she is faced with two conflicting attitudes within
herself: overconfidence and fear. It is essential to approach your dual responsibilities with as practical a plan
as possible in order to avoid not only fear of failure but
the superwoman syndrome.

The superwoman syndrome. You may feel that you
are being tested by your employer, your spouse, your baby
and even yourself to prove that you can combine work
and mothering. This sets up the superwoman syndrome,
in which you try to do everything, ultimately resulting in
fatigue, stress, overload, resentment and anger.

Once again, as during your pregnancy, the key to easing
the transition from pregnant worker to working mother is
planning. Try to think about your postpartum plans toward the end of your pregnancy so that you have a better
start on reentry planning before the baby arrives. Now is
the time to consider the pros and cons of breast feeding
and how this might work into your schedule. For the
working mother this may be a special problem. Can you
breast-feed on the job? Does your office have child-care

facilities or permit new mothers to have their babies with them at work? Will your employer permit you to return home if you live close by your office to breast-feed the baby during the early postpartum period if you return to work before your breast-feeding days have ended? How do you feel about expressing your breast milk into a bottle and leaving it with your caretaker so that she can feed the baby? Think about what is most important to you regarding your work, and plan accordingly. It may require a little creative compromise. You may have to place some limits on yourself, and take time away from child and/or job. But if you are a high-potential employee, you won't risk much. Work and mothering can be combined, but you may have to alter your perceptions toward one of these in order to carry off both responsibilities. You may as well accept the fact that you cannot go full tilt at both unless you have full-time, live-in help, are extremely wealthy, have a husband who will share responsibilities all the time and have a job located five minutes from the house. There are few of us who have everything. So you will probably have to compromise a bit.

Many women—several of them prominent feminists and scholars—are beginning to come to the same conclusions as that expressed by a Tennessee school administrator: "I really don't think that a woman has to live the same way men live. It's very hard to come to that decision when you don't have any role models. The only role models I had were male, and very often I felt there was something wrong with me because I wasn't like them. I don't feel that way anymore, and all of that came together in my mind when I was pregnant and had to decide what I was going to do with my work and my baby."

The fact that you are committed to working illustrates one aspect of your confidence, but you must also respect your qualities as a woman. And if you are planning to combine work and mothering successfully, you must respect this fact and deal with it rather than ignore it.

The fact that women have much to offer as women rather than as emulations of the male model is the subject of a recent book, *In Transition: How Feminism, Sexual*

*Liberation, and the Search for Self-fulfillment Have
Altered Our Lives,* by Judith Bardwick, one of the fore-
most authorities in the United States on the psychology of
women. Bardwick, associate dean and professor of psychology at the University of Michigan, explained in a
personal interview that when a woman has clearly demonstrated her competence, it becomes much easier to
come to terms with her values as a woman. She said that
as more women entered the work world, and as their
presence became normalized, there would eventually be
greater acceptance of women as individual contributors
rather than as characterizations as a class.

Bardwick told an anecdote of her attendance at a fac-
ulty meeting where several issues were being debated.
She had to leave early to pick up her daughter from
drama class, and excused herself from the meeting. "A
few years ago, I would have made up an excuse about
having a business meeting, but I no longer feel that I
have to do that. When I left the meeting I said I had to
pick up my daughter, and explained. 'This mother is
leaving.'"

You as a working woman with a child have a lot to
offer to both your job and your offspring, and with a little
planning and compromise you will succeed in both roles.
You do not have to play the same role as your male
colleagues. And you will not fail because you will be
calling your own shots.

DEALING WITH GUILT

Probably the most difficult part of being a working mother is dealing with guilt. The old rules that say a mother
belongs with the child are very strong, and there are
practical realities to carry off successfully the dual roles
of worker and mother. You will need confidence to function with as little guilt as possible, especially in coping
with adverse comments from those around you. You will
need to be secure in the belief that your child-care arrangement is the best possible, and that you have made
plans for backup care if an emergency should arise.

Here are some of the comments most frequently made
to working mothers, and our suggestions for your answers:

"Don't you think your child suffers because you are not home?"
"No."

"Don't you miss your child?"
"Of course."

"You're missing your baby's best moments."
"I'll see the repeat performance."

"Does your child know who his mother is?"
"Does yours?"

"I don't know how you can do it."
"I don't know how *you* can do it."

You will receive many comments from others, and you can answer them directly without much explanation. Those who are criticizing you may be questioning their own decision, whatever that may be.

As for child care, you have probably thought about it during your pregnancy. If not, before you do anything, determine what you really want in a caretaker. Do you want a baby-care person or a maid to clean your house? It is rare to find a person who is both things. A key criterion in hiring that person should be reliability, and one way of ascertaining how reliable that person is may be to ask for a year's commitment. Hours are also essential. Some caretakers are specialists. Some will take care only of newborns; others prefer an older child. Make sure that you are clear in your own mind what your requirements are.

Sources for caretakers are

- Agencies

- Friends, including colleagues who are working parents

- Student nurses, for intermediate and temporary baby sitting with your infant

- Advertisements (be specific in your wording, giving hours, wages, whether full-time or part-time and number of children)

- Day-care centers (check them out personally and ask lots of questions)

Once you have made your child-care arrangements, you should be aware that your anxiety will not diminish. You may have to have a backup plan in case of contingency. Therefore, try a few game plans regarding your baby and your caretaker. Write down your worst fears. Try to anticipate what you would do if:

- *Your child became sick.* What is sick? Is it a cold—or a broken arm? Must you be there? Does your caretaker know where to take your child in an emergency? Does your caretaker drive? If not, how would she or he handle an emergency situation?

  Where is the nearest hospital? Can your child be admitted without you? (In many instances he or she may not be admitted without your signature.) Does your pediatrician have privileges at the nearest hospital?

  Does your caretaker have emergency numbers—your office, your mate's office, neighbor, doctor, hospital, your health insurance policy company, police, fire, poison control center—all listed next to your telephone or written on one list to be taken to your caretaker's house?

- *Your caretaker either didn't show up—or said she could no longer care for your child.* Do you have an emergency plan or backup person? Will your husband split baby-care responsibilities while you are looking for a new person so that you can work?

  Ask yourself why this person left in the first place. Was it for a better job? Higher wages? Or because you did not make it clear what the requirements of the job were?

- *You have to go out of town and your husband is away; your caretaker will not (or is not able to) care for the child overnight.* Either take the baby with you—and hire someone at your destination (there are many nursing agencies in virtually every city)—or call a local agency for a temporary replacement. This is a temporary solution, and you should think of it in that sense. You should be aware of agencies in your community that may offer such services.

  A neighbor or family member can certainly be called upon in an emergency, but don't abuse your friends or relatives with many last-minute drop-off requests.

One other point should be made with regard to child care: Your spouse may tell you that your entire salary is going for child care, other help and taxes, so you should stay home, since there is no financial benefit gained by your working. Think seriously about this argument. There may be a point here, but would you be happy at home all day? If not, tell your spouse and yourself that at least you are keeping your foot in the door, and you enjoy being out of the house and at work. This period of time will pass, and as the baby gets older you will require less help and can move on to another stage—concerning child care and financial needs.

If you feel that you really would miss a work environment, ask your husband if he fully understands the enjoyment you receive from your job. Ask him how he would feel giving up his job to stay home with a newborn. Explain that you will be a better companion because of your dual job and mothering interests—and mention the fact that you may lose your competitive salary momentum should you drop out of the labor force and have to face reentry (and new salary negotiations) at some point in the future.

Not Being a Working Mother Also Involves Compromise

If you worked prior to becoming pregnant, people may ask when you will be returning to work, because today it is fashionable to have a job. The working woman makes good newspaper copy. No one wants to read about the mother of the year.

Many women want to stay home with their children, however, and for those who do, guilt should not be part of the arrangement. It takes an enormous amount of energy and effort to raise a child, and if you do it well it is a very difficult job. Women who want the job and involvement of running a home and caring for their children will probably work harder than those with a full-time job outside the home.

Thus there is no reason to feel guilty about your decision to be a career homemaker. Nevertheless, when others ask you what you do you may feel a twinge of guilt. Reply that your chosen occupation is motherhood, and that you are pleased that you have accepted the job.

The view from Sesame Street is not always a cheery one, however, and although you may be delighted to be a career mother—either on a long-term basis or for the short-term duration of a maternity leave—there are many problems common to those of you who elect to stay out of the labor force. In order to help you combat frustration, isolation and lack of adult contacts, we will offer a few suggestions.

Make sure your spouse understands what it is like to be home all day with an infant. He may underestimate what you've been doing, which in turn may cause a great deal of frustration to build up inside you.

Your husband may come home at the end of the day, expecting to see you shining and bright for him, and instead find you looking haggard and acting snappish, your shoulders covered with drool. Instead of sympathizing with you, he most likely will ask what you have been doing all day—and why life with a baby should be so difficult. Well, it *is* difficult, and make sure he understands why and how. Leave *him* with the baby for a full day as soon as you have resumed your strength.

It is essential that your husband understand the emotional and physical experiences you are undergoing, especially in the immediate postpartum period, when the baby is making round-the-clock demands.

How to Break the Cycle of Frustration and Isolation

The baby has become a part of your lives, but for the first six months or so you will probably be so caught up with your new mothering activities that you won't notice that your own emotional needs may have been neglected. In order to maintain your stability, you should try and get out of the house at least once a day.

You can become a hermit and let your life revolve around your child, but you may then become emotionally dependent on that child, which will have grievous effects on your life. If you do not make an effort to get out, you may lose contact with the outside world, resentment may build up and it may transfer to your spouse and/or your child. Avoid this at all costs and get out—even if only to go to the grocery store.

If you do not have help, try a mother's helper. This will force you to schedule time for yourself. Mother's helpers are usually high school students who take care of a child from the time they come home from school until the dinner hour. If there are no young men or women available in your neighborhood, ask around or place an ad in your local newspaper. You might also call the job placement service at your local high school.

If you are uncertain about leaving a new person with your baby, then let the helper stay in the house or same room with the baby—and you disappear into another section of the house. This will build up your confidence in your helper being alone with the baby for an hour or two.

The goal at this point is *not* regular help or a baby-sitting service—it is to provide a break for you from your regular baby-care schedule and the demands the child is making on you. Even if you do nothing but retire to another room to read, sew, prepare dinner or visit with a friend, you will be refreshed and discover that the few dollars expended on your helper will be one of the best small investments you have ever made.

Other ways of breaking the routine are the following:

- Let your husband stay with the baby for a few hours, either on a weekend or at night while you go out to a movie or shopping.

- Meet a friend for lunch or dinner.

- Go shopping alone.

- Meet your spouse for a quiet lunch.

If it is absolutely impossible to find help during the week, try taking the baby with you to different places you would like to visit, such as a museum or zoo. This will offer a change in scenery for both of you.

Finding New Friends

Somewhere around the sixth week, when the baby begins to follow a more regular routine and you are a bit more rested, you may discover that you lack adult contact. If you have previously worked, you may discover that you do not know anyone in your neighborhood because you weren't around much before. Or if you have moved to a new area, you won't know anyone either.

Where you live determines how you find new friends, and presuming you would like to meet a few new people (preferably with small children), here are a few ideas how:

- Walk around your neighborhood with your baby. You will be amazed how many mothers appear when you are out with a baby. They may also be looking for new people, and most are very open and friendly because they are concerned about their children having contact with other children as well. They may not turn out to be great friends, but the exposure to other adults with small children will be very helpful to you now.

- Get involved in organizational work. Try to determine what activities might interest you, and begin asking around to see what is available in your area. There are usually church-related, community, political, social and art organizations. Some have volunteer activities; some require a small fee for joining.

  Go to a few "meets and greets," and see if any interest you. If they do, arrange for help or take the baby with you. Many organizations offer baby sitting or child care during their meeting or activity times. You may meet some people with whom you share common interests, and it will give you some new adult contact.

- Join a sports group. Even if you are not very athletic, think about what sport interests you. Join a bowling or tennis league or take lessons. This is a great way to meet other women and couples—and out of this should come at least a few with small children.

- Call a few of the participants in your prepared childbirth class and suggest getting together.

- Call your pediatrician, explain that you would like to meet a few other mothers in your area, and see if he or she has any suggestions.

- Join your local YMCA, YWHA or other association. Many have adult and children's activities. It is up to you to determine what you would like to participate in.

From these initial beginnings your circle of friends should grow. It will not happen overnight, but it will be a start toward getting you more involved in the world around you and making you less dependent on the baby for conversation and socialization.

Once you become accustomed to your new addition and more relaxed about your role, you will see how easy it is to let the baby revolve around you instead of the other way around.

POSTPARTUM RELATIONSHIP WITH YOUR SPOUSE

No matter how wonderful your relationship with your husband has been during your pregnancy or how supportive he has been during labor and delivery, after the baby actually becomes a part of your household some changes may occur.

The baby makes enormous emotional demands on you. It cries, it wants to be fed, held and changed, and it cries again. You will be tired and anxious and there will be times when your spouse will simply not be aware of these new demands made on you. He may expect the same relationship with you as before, and be very surprised and resentful when your relationship begins to change. Your husband may feel that he is losing "center stage" in your attention.

A new baby requires adjustment and it is up to you to help ease that adjustment.

Whether you work or not, there will be some dual responsibilities required of both you and your spouse during the postpartum period. One way to ease this transition is to work out a parenting scheme.

Develop a system for sharing responsibilities. In this way you will reduce the tension and resentment that often builds when you are exhausted from dealing with a new set of emotional demands.

Depending on your particular situation, whether you plan to return to work, whether you have help, or whether you have elected to stay home, sit down and draw up a list with your husband about what must be done each week.

Include the normal household tasks, such as cooking,

cleaning and shopping, but also take into consideration certain obligations, such as business appointments your husband might have or perhaps even a Saturday morning two-hour work stint to catch up.

Then look over the list, estimate the time required for each activity and divide up the responsibilities. **MAKE SURE YOU INCLUDE BABY CARE IN THE LIST.**

You will probably want to devote your major tasks to the baby, so let your spouse be the backup. Draw up a shopping list, and let him stop at the store on the way home from the office.

Let your mate take the animals to the vet for their shots. Let him do the banking activities—or bank by mail. Either let your mate take the baby to the doctor for one of his first checkups or insist that he come with you.

Insist that he help you, and some of these duties may carry over into the postpartum period.

When you feel stronger and a bit more relaxed, you will probably want to use these errands as excuses to get out if you don't work and as weekend outings if you do work.

With a little planning, the transition period may be a little easier for both of you.

In the words of one of the women we interviewed, "Once the baby comes, life is never the same, and the moments you have spent with that man as a twosome will never come again. You don't have them on vacation because your mind—at least my mind—is at home with the baby. I don't want to go away on vacation for more than five days because I miss the baby, yet I don't want to take him with us because we need some time together alone. Life is never going to be the same. Whether life would change anyway without the child, I don't know. I can't say. But I wouldn't want it any differently."

POSTSCRIPT

The New Pregnancy is not only a state of activity, it is a state of mind as well. For you who have children today, this state of mind may have more effect on your life than the pregnancy itself.

What this means is that the way you live and the way you look at yourself and your pregnancy may well change the way you look at other aspects of your life.

Your Job

If you have worked, you may not want to give up your job or career to concentrate on childrearing. You may want to combine both activities and may discover that this entails compromise.

A child does add a complexity to your life simply because it presents another person's needs to consider, but with an enthusiastic outlook and flexible attitude you may discover that it *can* be done.

To achieve these dual roles, however, you may have to educate your spouse about the sharing of responsibilities that a two-worker family with children often requires. Parenting is a dual responsibility and should not fall solely on the mother.

It will affect your job, since occasionally a parent must stay home with a child because of illness or other reasons; but it should not automatically be assumed that *you* should

213

be the one to give up a day's work. After all, you may
have just as much to lose by your absence from work as
your spouse does.

The New Pregnancy may also encourage employers to
reassess and tailor some of their career slots to fit the
unique attributes of the career women who want to accommodate both their jobs and their children. Flexible
hours, rotating job duties and part-time or shared employment positions are some of the ways employers can
maximize the use of employees who want to continue to
work after childbirth, but who may require somewhat
more flexibility during the first few years of early childhood. In turn, you may find that your employer may
require higher productivity from you as part of the trade-
off that enables you to spend more time with your child.

The New Pregnancy has implications for other women
who follow you in the work force. With a continued trend
toward an increase in female labor force participation and
an accompanying decrease in women stopping work solely
due to pregnancy, the working mother inevitably will
constitute a larger portion of the total work force. They
may thus exert more pressure on employers for better
maternity leave, adequate temporary disability coverage
and more equitable health insurance.

Ultimately the increasing numbers of working mothers
(and working fathers) may push Congress toward a re-
thinking of public policies regarding social security and
income tax laws to reflect the realities of the two-income
childbearing family.

Your Child Care

One of the biggest concerns of the working parent today
is adequate child care. It is a common problem. More
and better day-care facilities or caretaker programs may
well be required to serve the needs of the working mother and the demands of young children. This in turn will
make it easier to nurture children.

On a broad social basis, if the U.S. population is ultimately to replace itself, then the concept of a working
pregnancy (and working motherhood) must be acceptable,
and adequate child care must be available.

Your Family

The growing presence of more women in the labor force is causing society to revise many sexual stereotypes, and motherhood is no longer the bottom-line role for all women. This revision is forcing more men to participate in the family unit from the prenatal period onward, and may lead to a stronger family environment in the future.

In addition, the new attitudes toward pregnancy and childbearing may provide an opportunity for reevaluating career situations, such as extensive travel and job transfers, which formerly encouraged disruption rather than stability of the family situation.

Yourself

Most of all the New Pregnancy means a new way of looking at yourself. It means questioning the attitude that there is only one role for a woman and only one way to have and raise a child.

The key word is *choice*. The New Pregnancy allows that choice to be yours and puts *you* in control of your future.

It is up to *you* to make the most of this very special time. You *can* have a successful and active pregnancy and set the stage for the years ahead if you

- Think and act as if pregnancy is an aspect of your life, not your whole life.

- Question any myth or attitude that says that you are apart from the rest of humanity just because you are pregnant.

- Stop yourself any time you think, "I can't do that, I'm pregnant" —and get the facts.

- Show confidence in the way that you are living, and have a plan so that you will know what you will be doing two months, six months or even a year from now.

- Develop a support team so that you will have the kind of encouragement to help you thrive.

- Set an example—show other women that an active pregnancy is possible and satisfying. Every obstacle you bypass will help others.

- Enjoy your pregnancy. Childbearing can be one of the greatest experiences of your life.

APPENDIX

Resources to Tap:
Where to Go If You Have
a Problem

RESOURCE

USEFULNESS

*American College of
Obstetricians and
Gynecologists*
Resource Center
One East Wacker Dr.
Suite 2700
Chicago, Ill. 60601

ACOG can supply selection
of board-certified
obstetricians and specialists
in your area; has a selection
of free public-information
pamphlets; and sets the
standards within the
profession.

*Directory of Medical
Specialties*
Marquis Who's Who
200 East Ohio St.
Chicago, Ill. 60611

The so-called blue book
can usually be found in
libraries. It lists board-
certified obstetricians,
giving their backgrounds. It
does not, however, list
obstetricians who may meet
many qualifications of
ACOG, but have not yet
taken or passed the
necessary examination. The

RESOURCE	**USEFULNESS**
	blue book is useful to check out physicians in your community, and may help in the selection of a pediatrician.
Physician's Desk Reference Medical Economics Co. Oradell, N.J. 07649	The PDR lists a wide variety of medications. Look under "contraindications during pregnancy."
American College of Nurse-Midwives 1012 14th St., N.W. Washington, D.C. 20005	Can supply names of nurse-midwifery services in your area and answer questions.
International Childbirth Education Association P.O. Box 20048 Minneapolis, Minn. 55420	This umbrella organization covers groups dedicated to family-centered maternity care and a prepared childbirth experience. Its consumer group holds many workshops throughout the country, and sponsors newsletters and a variety of publications. *Note*. There are many different organizations and philosophies about methods of prepared childbirth. The ICEA is widely known and respected, and is an excellent initial source of information. ICEA maintains a mail order "book center" of current books, reprints, pamphlets and so on about every phase of the

RESOURCE	USEFULNESS
	pregnancy, childbirth and child-care experience. Also publishes *Bookmarks,* a newsletter offering book lists and reviews. One item to look for: *The Pregnancy Patient's Bill of Rights/ The Pregnant Patient's Responsibilities.*
C-Sec. Inc. 66 Christopher Rd. Waltham, Mass. 02154	C-Sec offers information on and referral for the self-help approach to dealing with the cesarean birth experience.
COPE (Coping with the Overall Pregnancy Experience) 37 Clarendon St. Boston, Mass. 02116	These two groups are good examples of the self-help approach of people going through similar experiences, and they offer group work and information resources.
Mothers' Center Family Service Association United Methodist Church Nelson and Cherry Sts. Hicksville, N.Y. 11801	They can also give you some ideas about trying their helpful approach in your community if nothing is already available to you.
National Association of Parents & Professionals for Safe Alternatives in Childbirth (NAPSAC) P.O. Box 1307 Chapel Hill, N.C. 27514	This is a major source for information about home births and other alternate maternity-care approaches. Its Institute for Childbirth and Family Research has reprints of research reports

RESOURCE	USEFULNESS
	relevant to its area of interest, which is not as fully explored by traditional medicine.
March of Dimes Birth Defects Foundation Box 2000 White Plains, N.Y. 10602	The Foundation offers a wide variety of free literature about pregnancy and precautions regarding birth defects. Local chapters are ready sources of information. The Foundation is a major force on behalf of research to prevent birth defects and in educating medical professionals.
Psychological Consultation Service for Parents and Prospective Parents c/o Zuckerberg 36 Montgomery Place Brooklyn, N.Y. 11215	Professionals as well as individuals seeking information about the emotional aspects of pregnancy and sources of aid will find this fairly unique service of use.
National Women's Health Network 224 7th Street Washington, D.C. 20006	The Network offers its members information and updates on all health issues important to women with maternal-child health a special concern. Membership fee is low, and adjusted to income.

ACOG-NIOSH Guidelines

This is a copy of the guidelines prepared by ACOG-NIOSH to aid medical personnel in determining aspects of your work environment which may prove harmful to you. You may want to use these guidelines to offer information about your work environment to your health support team.

QUESTIONS FOR OCCUPATIONAL HISTORY

This format may be used for assembling data about the employed patient and her partner to supplement the usual obstetrical history and home information.

1. TYPE AND PLACE OF WORK:

	Patient	Male Partner
Job title:		
Employer:		
Union:		
Supervisor:		
Occupational Health Staff:		

This identifies the patient and persons to contact for further information. It is intended to augment the usual identifying and demographic data with information about the job setting

Information about the male partner is important if he is a potential carrier of toxic substances or infection.

2. WORK SCHEDULE:

Inquire about days worked, hours worked, schedule changes, frequency and amount of overtime, rest periods and breaks, frequency and regulation of work flow.

This establishes the duration of work and the regularity of the work schedule. If rest periods are taken, ask whether these are on schedule or taken as needed. Adverse effects often can be obviated by altering the work schedule or changing the work/rest ratio. The flexibility of work flow is often important: can the woman set her pace, or is it dictated by a process like assembly-line work? Are there busy and slack times or is the pace steady?

3. AMENITIES:

Inquire about lavatory, rest areas, food and drink, access to emergency care.

This establishes the availability and accessibility of amenities that may be of special importance to pregnant workers. Can she go to the lavatory as needed? Is there a place to rest? To dine? Can arrangements be made for additional meals or rest periods as advised?

4. PHYSICAL WORK:

Inquire about the nature of the activity, particularly sitting, standing, and other activities (such as walking, bending, climbing).

This establishes duration of continuous activity in hours and minutes, and the frequency per period in which these activities are performed.

Continuous sitting may affect lower spine and venous return. Type of chair and availability of footstool are important. Bar-type chairs may be used to relieve the standing worker.

Inquire about the nature of the load handled by the worker.

This establishes the force (weight) required, size and shape, and type of handling such as lifting or pulling.

Inquire about task characteristics, including the balance and coordination required, risks of falling, task complexity, agility required by moving machinery or objects, sudden starts and stops, belts and harnesses.

This establishes information about any possible hazards related to the possibility of falling, either as a result of impaired balance or dizziness in pregnancy, or because of use of ladders or precarious positions. The risk of being struck or of the abdomen being impinged between spine and an external object is important.

5. ENVIRONMENTAL CHARACTERISTICS:

Inquire about exposure to important environmental factors such as
  —climate, temperature
  —barometric pressure
  —noise, vibration
  —radiation
  —biologic agents
  —airborne dusts, fumes, vapors
  —chemicals
  —special job characteristics

This establishes exposure to toxic factors in the environment. Each of these is discussed in more detail with respect to specific reproductive and systemic effects elsewhere in this document.

Note the intensity—if possible in actual measurements—and the duration of the exposure.

Also note any special job characteristics that may reduce or increase exposures: occlusive garments, ventilation, close quarters, isolation, available emergency equipment or transportation, emotional stress.

Source: Reprinted from *Guidelines on Pregnancy and Work*, American College of Obstetricians and Gynecologists, 1977.

Examples of Women's Occupational Exposures

The following tables include examples of occupations in which a high proportion of women are employed. Some of the occupations with a very large female work force may also be considered among the most hazardous.

	1970	1960	Increase
Sewers and stitchers	812,716	534,258	34%
Registered nurses	807,359	567,884	30%
Nursing aides, orderlies, and so on	609,022	485,383	20%
Assemblers	454,611	270,769	40%
Hairdressers and cosmetologists	424,873	267,050	37%
Checkers, examiners, inspectors (manufacturing)	327,530	215,066	34%
Packers and wrappers	314,067	262,935	16%

Some of the typical occupational exposures are listed below. Note that not all the substances included are referred to in *Guidelines on Pregnancy and Work*, published by the ACOG. Specific information about the toxicity of any particular substance can be obtained from the resources listed on pages 227–37.

OCCUPATION   EXPOSURES

Textile and Related Operatives (see note)

Textile operatives	Raw cotton dust, noise, synthetic fiber dusts, formaldehyde, heat, dyes, flame retardants, asbestos
Sewers and stitchers	Cotton and synthetic fiber dusts, noise, formaldehyde, organic solvents, flame retardants, asbestos

OCCUPATION	EXPOSURES
Upholsterers	See Sewers and Stitchers
Hospital/Health Personnel	
Registered nurses, aides, orderlies	Anesthetic gases, ethylene oxide, X-ray radiation, alcohol, infectious diseases, puncture wounds
Dental hygienists	X-ray radiation, mercury, ultrasonic noise, anesthetic gases
Laboratory workers (clinical and research)	Wide variety of toxic chemicals, including carcinogens, mutagens and teratogens, X-ray radiation
Electronics Assemblers	Lead, tin, antimony, trichloroethylene, methylene chloride, expoxy resins, methyl ethyl ketone
Hairdressers and Cosmetologists	Hair spray resins (polyvinylpyrrolidone), aerosol propellants (freons), halogenated hydrocarbons, hair dyes, solvents of nail polish, benzyl alcohol, ethyl alcohol, acetone
Cleaning Personnel	
Launderers	Soaps, detergents, enzymes, heat, humidity, industrially contaminated clothing

Note: Some specific chemicals encountered in these occupations are benzene, toluene, trichloroethylene, perchloroethylene, chloroprene, styrene, carbon disulfide.

OCCUPATION	EXPOSURES
Dry cleaners	Perchloroethylene, trichloroethylene, stoddard solvent (naphtha), benzene, industrially contaminated clothing
Photographic Processors	Caustics, iron salts, mercuric chloride, bromides, iodides, pyrogallate acid and silver nitrate
Plastic Fabricators	Acrylonitrile, phenolformaldehydes, ureaformaldehydes, hexamethylenetetramine, acids, alkalies, peroxide, vinyl chloride, polystyrene, vinylidene chloride
Domestics	Solvents, hydrocarbons, soaps, detergents, bleaches, alkalies
Transportation Operatives	Carbon monoxide, polynuclear aromatics, lead and other combustion products of gasoline, vibration, physical stresses
Sign Painters and Letterers	Lead oxide, lead chromate pigments, epichlorohydrin, titanium dioxide, trace metals, xylene, toluene
Clerical Personnel	Physical stresses, poor illumination, trichloroethylene, carbon tetrachloride and various

OCCUPATION	EXPOSURES
	other cleaners, asbestos in air-conditioning
Opticians and Lens Grinders	Coal tar pitch volatiles, iron oxide dust solvents, hydrocarbons
Printing Operatives	Ink mists, 2-nitropropane, methanol, carbon tetrachloride, methylene chloride, lead, noise, hydrocarbon solvents, trichloroethylene, toluene, benzene, trace metals

Source: Reprinted from *Guidelines on Pregnancy and Work*, American College of Obstetricians and Gynecologists, 1977.

Occupational Hazards Resources

The following is a list of resources to tap for information and questions about occupational hazards:

National Institute for Occupational Safety and Health

NATIONAL HEADQUARTERS

Parklawn Bldg.
5600 Fishers Ln.
Rockville, Md. 20857

CINCINNATI OFFICE

Robert A. Taft Laboratories
4676 Columbia Pky.
Cincinnati, Ohio 45226

APPALACHIAN CENTER

Appalachian Center for Occupational Safety and Health (ACOSH)
944 Chestnut Ridge Rd.
Morgantown, W.V. 26505

REGIONAL OFFICES

Region I: Connecticut, Maine, Massachusetts, New Hampshire, Rhode Island, Vermont

Regional Consultant,
NIOSH DHEW, Region I
Government Center (JFK
Fed. Bldg.)
Boston, Mass. 02203
617 223-6668

*Region II: New Jersey,
New York, Puerto Rico,
Virgin Islands*

Regional Consultant,
NIOSH DHEW, Region
II—Fed. Bldg.
26 Federal Plaza
New York, N.Y. 10007
212 264-2485

*Region III: Delaware,
District of Columbia,
Maryland, Pennsylvania,
Virginia, West Virginia*

Regional Consultant,
NIOSH DHEW, Region III
P.O. Box 13716
Philadelphia, Pa. 19101
215 596-6716

*Region IV: Alabama,
Florida, Georgia, Kentucky,
Mississippi, North
Carolina, South Carolina,
Tennessee*

Regional Consultant,
NIOSH DHEW, Region IV
101 Marietta Tower, Ste. 502
Atlanta, Ga. 30303
404 221-2396

*Region V: Illinois, Indiana,
Michigan, Minnesota,
Ohio, Wisconsin*

Regional Consultant,
NIOSH DHEW, Region V
300 South Wacker Dr.
Chicago, Ill. 60607
312 886-3881

*Region VI: Arkansas,
Louisiana, New Mexico,
Oklahoma, Texas*

Regional Consultant,
NIOSH DHEW, Region VI
1200 Main Tower Bldg.
Rm. 1700-A
Dallas, Tex. 75202
214 767-3916

*Region VII: Iowa, Kansas,
Missouri, Nebraska*

Regional Consultant,
NIOSH DHEW, Region VII
601 East 12th St.
Kansas City, Mo. 64106
816 374-5332

*Region VIII: Colorado,
Montana, Utah, Wyoming,
North Dakota, South
Dakota*

Regional Consultant,
NIOSH DHEW/PHS/
Prevention—Region VIII
11037 Federal Bldg.
Denver, Colo. 82094
303 837-3979

*Region IX: Arizona,
California, Hawaii, Nevada*

Regional Consultant,
NIOSH DHEW, Region IX
50 United Nations Plaza
Rm. 231
San Francisco, Calif. 94102
415 556-3781

*Region X: Alaska, Idaho,
Oregon, Washington*

Regional Consultant,
NIOSH DHEW, Region X
1321 Second Ave. (Arcade
Bldg.)
Seattle, Wash. 98101
206 442-0530

Occupational Safety and Health Administration

HEADQUARTERS

Occupational Safety and
Health Administration
U.S. Department of Labor
200 Constitution Ave., N.W.
Washington, D.C. 20210

REGIONAL OFFICES

*Region I: Connecticut,
Maine, Massachusetts,
New Hampshire, Rhode
Island, Vermont*

U.S. Department of
Labor—OSHA
16-18 North St.
1 Dock Square Bldg.
4th floor
Boston, Mass. 02109
617 223-6710

*Region II: New Jersey, New
York, Puerto Rico, Virgin
Islands, Canal Zone*

Regional Administrator
U.S. Department of Labor—
OSHA
1515 Broadway (1 Astor
Plaza)
Rm. 3445
New York, N.Y. 10036
212 944-3426

*Region III: Delaware,
District of Columbia,
Maryland, Pennsylvania,
Virginia, West Virginia*

Regional Administrator
U.S. Department of Labor
—OSHA
Gateway Bldg.—Suite 2100
3535 Market St.
Philadelphia, Pa. 19104
215 596-1201

*Region IV: Alabama,
Florida, Georgia, Kentucky,
Mississippi, North
Carolina, Tennessee*

Regional Administrator
U.S. Department of Labor—
OSHA
1375 Peachtree St., N.E.
Suite 587
Atlanta, Ga. 30367
404 881-3573

*Region V: Illinois, Indiana,
Minnesota, Ohio, Wisconsin*

Regional Administrator
U.S. Department of Labor—
OSHA
32nd Floor—Rm. 3244
230 South Dearborn St.
Chicago, Ill. 60604
312 353-2220

*Region VI: Arkansas,
Louisiana, New Mexico,
Oklahoma, Texas*

Regional Administrator
U.S. Department of Labor—
OSHA
555 Griffin Square Bldg.
Rm. 602
Dallas, Tex. 75202
214 767-4731

*Region VII: Iowa, Kansas,
Missouri, Nebraska*

Regional Administrator
U.S. Department of Labor—
OSHA
911 Walnut St.—Rm. 3000
Kansas City, Mo. 64106
816 374-5861

*Region VIII: Colorado,
Montana, North Dakota,
South Dakota, Utah,
Wyoming*

Regional Administrator
U.S. Department of Labor—
OSHA
Federal Bldg.
Rm. 1554
1961 Stout St.
Denver, Colo. 80294
303 837-3883

*Region IX: California,
Arizona, Nevada, Hawaii,
American Samoa, Guam,
Trust Territory of the
Pacific Islands*

Regional Administrator
U.S. Department of Labor—
OSHA
11349 Federal Bldg.
450 Golden Gate Ave.
P.O. Box 36017
San Francisco, Calif. 94102
415 556-0586

*Region X: Alaska, Idaho,
Oregon, Washington*

Regional Administrator
U.S. Department of Labor—
OSHA
Federal Office Bldg., Rm.
6003
909 First Ave.
Seattle, Wash. 98174
206 442-5930

State Designated Agencies

Alabama

Commissioner
Alabama Department of
Labor
600 Administrative Bldg.
64 North Union St.
Montgomery, Ala. 36130
205 832-6270

Alaska

Commissioner
Alaska Department of
Labor
P.O. Box 1149
Juneau, Alaska 99811
907 465-2700

Arizona

Director
Industrial Commission on
Arizona
1601 W. Adams
P.O. Box 19070
Phoenix, Ariz. 85005
602 271-4411

Arkansas

Commissioner
Arkansas Department of
Labor
Capitol Hill Bldg.
Little Rock, Ark. 72201
501 371-1401

California

Secretary
Agriculture and Services
Agency
1220 N St., Rm. 409
Sacramento, Calif. 95814
916 445-1935

Colorado

Director
Colorado Division of Labor
Department of Labor and
Employment
1313 Sherman St.
Denver, Colo. 80203
303 892-3596

Connecticut

Commissioner
Department of Labor
200 Folly Brook Blvd.
Wethersfield, Conn. 06109
203 566-4384

Delaware

Secretary
Department of Labor
801 West St.
Wilmington, Del. 19801
302 571-2710

District of Columbia

Director
Minimum Wage and
Industrial Safety Board
Industrial Safety Division
Government of the District
of Columbia
2900 Newton St., N.E.
Washington, D.C. 20018
202 832-1230

Florida

Secretary
Department of Commerce
Division of Labor
510 Collins Bldg.
Tallahassee, Fl. 32304
904 488-3104

Georgia

Commissioner
Department of Labor
288 State Labor Bldg.
Atlanta, Ga. 30334
404 656-3011

Guam

Director
Division of Occupational
Safety
Department of Labor
Government of Guam
P.O. Box 884 (JSMP)
Agana, Guam 96910
777-9822

Hawaii

Director
Department of Labor
Industrial Relations
825 Mililani St.
Honolulu, Hawaii 96813
808 548-3151

Idaho

Commissioner
Department of Labor
317 Main St., Rm. 300
Boise, Idaho 83702
208 964-2327

Illinois

Director
Illinois Department of
Labor
160 North La Salle St.
Chicago, Ill. 60601
312 793-2800

Indiana

Commissioner
Indiana Division of Labor
Indiana State Office Bldg.
100 North Senate Ave.
Indianapolis, Ind. 46204
317 633-4473

Iowa

Commissioner
Bureau of Labor, State
House
East 7th & Court Ave.
Des Moines, Iowa 50319
515 281-3606

Kansas

Secretary
Department of Human
Resources
401 Topeka Ave.
Topeka, Kans. 66603
913 296-7474

Kentucky

Commissioner
Department of Labor
Capitol Plaza
Frankfort, Ky. 40601
502 564-3070

Louisiana

Commissioner
Louisiana Department of
Labor
P.O. Box 44063
Baton Rouge, La. 70804
504 389-5314

Maine

Commissioner
Department of Manpower
Affairs
State House
Augusta, Maine 04330
207 289-3814

Maryland

Commissioner
Division of Labor and
Industry
Department of Licensing
and Regulation
203 E. Baltimore St.
Baltimore, Md. 21202
301 383-2250

Massachusetts

Commissioner
Massachusetts Department
of Labor and Industries
Leverett Saltonstall Bldg.
Massachusetts Government
Center—11th Fl.
Boston, Mass. 02202
617 727-3454

Michigan

Director
Michigan Department of
Labor
309 N. Washington
Lansing, Mich. 48909
517 373-9600

Minnesota

Commissioner
State Department of
Labor and Industry
Space Center Bldg.—5th
Fl.
444 Lafayette Rd.
St. Paul, Minn. 55101
612 296-2342

Mississippi

State Health Officer
Mississippi State Board of
Health
P.O. Box 1700
Jackson, Miss. 39205
601 354-6646

Missouri

Commissioner
Missouri Department of
Labor and Industrial
Relations
Box 599
Jefferson City, Mo. 65101
314 751-2461

Montana

Administrator
Division of Workers'
Compensation
815 Front St.
Helena, Mont. 59601
406 449-2047

Nebraska

Commissioner
Department of Labor
P.O. Box 94600
State House Sta.
Lincoln, Nebr. 68509
402 475-8451

Nevada

Director
Department of Occupational
Safety and Health
Nevada Industrial
Commission
515 E. Musser St.
Carson City, Nev. 89701
702 885-5241

New Hampshire

Commissioner
State of New Hampshire
Department of Labor
(Occupational Safety)
1 Pillsbury St.
Concord, N.H. 03301
603 255-6611

New Jersey

Commissioner
Department of Labor and
Industry
John Fitch Plaza
Trenton, N.J. 08625
609 292-2323

New Mexico

Executive Director
Health and Social
Services Department
P.O. Box 2348
Santa Fe, N.M. 87501
505 827-2371

New York

Commissioner of Labor
State of New York
Two World Trade Center
New York, N.Y. 10047

North Carolina

Commissioner
North Carolina Department
of Labor
P.O. Box 27407
Raleigh, N.C. 27611
919 829-7166

North Dakota

Chairman
Workmen's Compensation
Bureau
Russell Bldg.
Highway 83 North
Bismarck, N. Dak. 58505
701 224-2700

Ohio

Chief
Division of Occupational
Safety and Health
Department of Industrial
Relations
2323 West Fifth Ave.,
Rm. 2380
Columbus, Ohio 43216
614 466-4124

Oklahoma

Commissioner
Oklahoma State Department
of Labor
State Capitol Bldg.
Oklahoma City, Okla.
73105
405 521-2461

Oregon

Board Chairman
Workmen's Compensation
Board
Labor and Industries Bldg.
Salem, Oreg. 97310
503 378-3311

Pennsylvania

Secretary
Department of Labor
and Industry
1700 Labor and Industry
Bldg.
Harrisburg, Pa. 17120
717 787-3157

Puerto Rico

Secretary of Labor
Department of Labor
Commonwealth of Puerto
Rico
414 Barbosa Ave.
San Juan, P.R. 00917
809 765-3030

Rhode Island

Director
Rhode Island Department
of Labor
235 Promenade St.
Providence, R.I. 20908
401 277-2741

South Carolina

Commissioner
Department of Labor
3600 Forest Dr.
P.O. Box 11329
Columbia, S.C. 29211
803 758-2851

South Dakota

Secretary of Health
Department of Health
Joe Foss Bldg.
Pierre, S. Dak. 57501
605 224-3361

Tennessee

Commissioner
Tennessee Department
of Labor
501 Union Bldg.
Nashville, Tenn. 37219
615 741-2582

Texas

Chief Bureau of
Environmental Health
Texas Department of Health
Resources
1100 West 49th St.
Austin, Tex. 78756
512 458-7542

Utah

Chairman
Utah Industrial Commission
350 East Fifth South
Salt Lake City, Utah 84111
801 533-6411

Vermont

Commissioner
Vermont Department of
Labor and Industries
Vermont State Office Bldg.
Montpelier, Vt. 05602
802 223-2311

Virginia

Commissioner
Department of Labor
and Industry
205 No. Fourth St.
Richmond, Va. 23219
804 786-2376

U.S. Virgin Islands

Commissioner of Labor
Virgin Islands Department
of Labor
Frederiksted, St. Croix
U.S. V.I. 00840
809 772-1315

Washington

Director
Department of Labor
and Industries
308 East Fourth Ave.
Olympia, Wash. 98501
206 753-6307

West Virginia

Commissioner
State Department of Labor
State Office Bldg. #6
1900 Washington St., E.
Charleston, W. Va. 25305
304 348-7890

Wisconsin

Chairman
Division of Safety and
Buildings
Department of Labor,
Industry and Human
Relations
201 East Washington
Ave.
P.O. Box 7946
Madison, Wis. 53707
608 266-1816; 3151 (R.R.)

Wyoming

Administrator
Occupational Health and
Safety Department
200 East Eighth Ave.
Cheyenne, Wyo. 82002
307 777-7786

Schools of Medicine

(Institutions with both Obstetrics-Gynecology and Occupational Medicine Programs or the equivalent)

University of Arizona
College of Medicine
Arizona Health Sciences
Center
Tucson, Ariz. 85724
602 882-6300

University of California at
Irvine
California College of
Medicine
Irvine, Calif. 92717
714 833-5838

University of Cincinnati
College of Medicine
231 Bethesda Ave.
Cincinnati, Ohio 45267
513 872-5491

Harvard Medical School
25 Shattuck St.
Boston, Mass. 02215
617 732-1000

Johns Hopkins
University
School of Medicine
720 Rutland Ave.
Baltimore, Md. 21205
301 955-5000

University of Illinois
College of Medicine
1853 West Polk St.
Chicago, Ill. 60612
312 996-2450

University of Michigan
Medical School
1335 Catherine St.
Ann Arbor, Mich. 48109
313 764-8173

University of Minnesota
Medical School
(Minneapolis)
145 Owre Hall
421 Delaware St., S.E.
Minneapolis, Minn. 55455
612 373-4570

New York University
School of Medicine
New York, N.Y. 10016
212 679-3200

University of North
Carolina at Chapel Hill
School of Medicine
Chapel Hill, N.C.
27514
919 966-4161

University of Texas
Health Science Center
at Houston
Medical School
P.O. Box 20708
Houston, Tex. 77025
713 792-2121

University of Utah
College of Medicine
50 North Medical Dr.
Salt Lake City, Utah
84132
801 581-7201

University of
Washington
School of Medicine
Seattle, Wash. 98195
206 543-1060

Yale University School of
Medicine
333 Cedar St.
New Haven, Conn.
06516
203 436-4771

Professional Associations

American Industrial
Hygiene Association
66 South Miller Rd.
Akron, Ohio 44313
216 836-9537

American Occupational
Medical Association
150 North Wacker Dr.
Chicago, Ill. 60606
312 782-2166

Members of the National Association of Insurance Commissioners

STATE	NAME AND TITLE	ADDRESS	TELEPHONE
Alabama	Tharpe Forrester Commissioner of Insurance	64 North Union St. Montgomery 36104	205 832-6140
Alaska	Kenneth C. Moore Director of Insurance	Pouch D Juneau 99811	907 465-2515
Arizona	J. Michael Low Director of Insurance	1601 West Jefferson Phoenix 85007	602 255-4862
Arkansas	William H. L. Woodyard III Insurance Commissioner	400-18 University Tower Bldg. Little Rock 72204	501 371-1325
California	Wesley J. Kinder Insurance Commissioner	600 South Commonwealth Los Angeles 90005	213 736-2551
Colorado	J. Richard Barnes Commissioner of Insurance	106 State Office Bldg. Denver 80203	303 839-3201
Connecticut	Joseph C. Mike Insurance Commissioner	Rm. 425, State Office Bldg. Hartford 06115	203 566-5275
Delaware	David Elliott Insurance Commissioner	21 The Green Dover 19901	302 678-4251
D.C.	James A. Montgomery (Acting) Superintendent of Insurance	614 H St., N.W., Suite 512 Washington 20001	202 727-1273

239

Members of the National Association of Insurance Commissioners

STATE	NAME AND TITLE	ADDRESS	TELEPHONE
Florida	Bill Gunter Insurance Commissioner	State Capitol Tallahassee 32304	904 488-3440
Georgia	Johnnie L. Caldwell Insurance Commissioner	238 State Capitol Atlanta 30334	404 656-2056
Guam	Ignacio C. Borja Insurance Commissioner	P.O. Box 2796 Agana 96910	
Hawaii	Tany S. Hong Insurance Commissioner	P.O. Box 3614 Honolulu 96811	808 548-7505
Idaho	Trent M. Woods Director of Insurance	700 West State St. Boise 83720	208 334-2250
Illinois	Philip R. O'Connor Director of Insurance	320 West Washington Springfield 62767	312 793-2420
Indiana	H. Pete Hudson Commissioner of Insurance	509 State Office Bldg. Indianapolis 46204	317 232-2385
Iowa	Bruce W. Foudree Commissioner of Insurance	State Office Bldg. Des Moines 50319	515 281-5705
Kansas	Fletcher Bell Commissioner of Insurance	State Office Bldg. Topeka 66612	913 296-3071

Kentucky	Daniel D. Briscoe Insurance Commissioner	151 Elkhorn Ct. Frankfort 40601	502 564-3630
Louisiana	Sherman A. Bernard Commissioner of Insurance	P.O. Box 44214 Baton Rouge 70804	504 342-5328
Maine	Theodore T. Briggs Superintendent of Insurance	State Office Building Augusta 04330	207 289-3141
Maryland	Edward J. Birrane, Jr. Insurance Commissioner	One South Calvert Bldg. Baltimore 21202	301 383-5690
Massachusetts	Michael J. Sabbagh Commissioner of Insurance	100 Cambridge St. Boston 02202	617 727-3333
Michigan	Nancy A. Baerwaldt Commissioner of Insurance	P.O. Box 30220 Lansing 48909	517 374-9724
Minnesota	Michael D. Markman Commissioner of Insurance	500 Metro Square Bldg. St. Paul 55101	612 296-6907
Mississippi	George Dale Commissioner of Insurance	P.O. Box 79 Jackson 39205	601 354-7711
Missouri	William Arthur Jones (Acting) Director of Insurance	P.O. Box 690 Jefferson City 65101	314 751-2451
Montana	Elmer V. Omholt Commissioner of Insurance	Mitchell Bldg. Helena 59601	406 449-2040

241

Members of the National Association of Insurance Commissioners

STATE	NAME AND TITLE	ADDRESS	TELEPHONE
Nebraska	Walter D. Weaver Director of Insurance	State Capitol Bldg., P.O. Box 94699, Lincoln 68509	402 471-2201 Ex. 238
Nevada	Donald W. Heath Insurance Commissioner	Nye Bldg. Carson City 89710	702 885-4270
New Hampshire	Frank E. Whaland Insurance Commissioner	169 Manchester Concord 03301	603 271-2261
New Jersey	James J. Sheeran Commissioner of Insurance	201 East State St. Trenton 08625	609 292-5363
New Mexico	Manuel A. Garcia, Jr. Superintendent of Insurance	Pera Building P.O. Drawer 1269 Santa Fe 87501	505 827-2451
New York	Albert B. Lewis Superintendent of Insurance	Two World Trade Center New York 10047	212 488-4124
No. Carolina	John R. Ingram Commissioner of Insurance	Dobbs Building P.O. Box 26387 Raleigh 27611	919 733-7343
No. Dakota	Byron Knutson Commissioner of Insurance	Capitol Bldg., 5th Fl. Bismarck 58505	701 224-2444
Ohio	Robert L. Ratchford Director of Insurance	2100 Stella Ct. Columbus 43215	614 466-2691

Oklahoma	Gerald Grimes Insurance Commissioner	408 Will Rogers Memorial Bldg. Oklahoma City 73105	405 521-2828
Oregon	Wilfred W. Fritz Insurance Commissioner	158-12th St., N.E. Salem 97310	503 378-4271
Pennsylvania	Michael L. Browne (Acting) Insurance Commissioner	Strawberry Sq., 13 & 14th Fls. Harrisburg 17120	717 787-5173
Puerto Rico	Rolando Cruz Commissioner of Insurance	P.O. Box 3508 San Juan 00904	809 724-6565
Rhode Island	Thomas J. Caldarone, Jr. Insurance Commissioner	100 North Main St. Providence 02903	401 277-2223
So. Carolina	John W. Lindsay Insurance Commissioner	2711 Middleburg Dr. Columbia 29204	803 758-3266
So. Dakota	Henry J. Lussen, Jr. Director of Insurance	Insurance Bldg. Pierre 57501	605 773-3563
Tennessee	John C. Neff Commissioner of Insurance	114 State Office Bldg. Nashville 37219	615 741-2241
Texas	E. J. Voorhis Commissioner of Insurance	1110 San Jacinto Blvd. Austin 78786	512 475-2273
Utah	Roger C. Day Commissioner of Insurance	326 South 5th East Salt Lake City 84102	801 533-5611

243

Members of the National Association of Insurance Commissioners

STATE	NAME AND TITLE	ADDRESS	TELEPHONE
Vermont	George A. Chaffee Commissioner of Insurance	State Office Bldg. Montpelier 05602	802 828-3301
Virginia	James W. Newman, Jr. Commissioner of Insurance	700 Blanton Bldg., P.O. Box 1157, Richmond 23209	804 786-3741
Virgin Islands	Henry A. Millin Commissioner of Insurance	P.O. Box 450 Charlotte Amalie St. Thomas 00801	809 774-2991
Washington	Dick Marquardt Insurance Commissioner	Insurance Bldg. AQ 21 Olympia 98504	206 753-7301
W. Virginia	Richard G. Shaw Insurance Commissioner	1800 Washington St., E. Charleston 25305	304 348-3386
Wisconsin	Susan Mitchell Commissioner of Insurance	123 West Washington Ave. Madison 53702	608 266-3585
Wyoming	John T. Langdon Insurance Commissioner	2424 Pioneer Cheyenne 82001	307 777-7401

Source: Reprinted courtesy of the National Association of Insurance Commissioners, Milwaukee, Wisconsin.

Filing a Complaint with an Outside Agency (Your State or Local Equal Employment Opportunity Office)

• *Accept the complaint procedure without illusion.* If you have been unable to settle your complaint in house, then you may want to go to an outside agency. If you opt for this route, then remember the guidelines presented in Chapter One, and face the process without illusion.

The complaint procedure is cumbersome and oftentimes costly, both in real dollars and in emotional expenditures. Accept these factors and recognize that you must become actively involved in pursuing your complaint through the system.

Remember that to file a complaint you need only believe that you were discriminated against.

If you prefer, you can file through an attorney or an interest group like NOW, or the EEOC can file the complaint for you.

One of the things in your favor is that employers do not want to be charged with a discrimination suit. Most do not want the annoyance, publicity, and potential costs of such a suit, so keep this in mind when approaching the complaint process.

• *Determine whether your state has a fair employment practice law (FEP), and begin at this level.* If it does, you must begin filing your claim through the appropriate state agency. You must check with your individual state, because not all states provide the same coverage and each state may treat the processing of a claim differently.

You must first find out which state agency enforces civil rights questions. The easiest way to do this is to look in your local telephone book under the state government listings. Some of the common listings for these agencies are Civil Rights Commission, Human Rights Commission, Human Relations Commission, and Fair Employment Practices Commission. If you cannot find any listing, call the general state government information number and say, "I think I've been discriminated against. Can you direct me to the proper agency?"

Not all states have these agencies, but most do. Many have toll-free numbers, regional or local offices. Call them, ask whether there is a state law forbidding discrimination based on pregnancy. Find out what the name, number or citation of the law is. Ask to talk to an official who handles these cases. Briefly explain your case and ask whether the state law will cover you.

You might also consider calling your state attorney general's office to say, "I want to know if there is a fair employment practice law in this state and where I can get a copy of it." Ask them to send you a copy so that you will be able to read what the law says.

Don't get discouraged if the people on the other end of the phone are rude, ignorant, put you on hold or transfer you a dozen times. This happens all the time. They are probably overworked and receive many calls from people like you. Be patient.

If your state does provide for such coverage and you have reason to believe you have been discriminated against on the basis of pregnancy, ask them to send you a charge form. If there is a local women's law project, ACLU office, legal rights office or NOW chapter in your community, you might also check with them to determine whether you may be eligible to file a charge and for advice on how to do it.

Even if your state has an FEP, some lawyers recommend filing a charge with the EEOC at the same time. The EEOC will "defer" or turn over your case to your state anyway if you are covered by a fair employment practice law, but it's added protection for you. (See pages 261–64 for a listing of EEOC district offices.)

● *Timing, timing, timing.* In any case, there are time limits for filing charges under both state and EEOC rules. Knowing these time limits is exceedingly important because of the way the process works. It takes time to gather background material in order to file a complaint, and it takes time to move a complaint through the bureaucracy.

You must file charges in writing with the EEOC within 180 days after the discriminatory act was committed. This does *not* mean 180 days after in-house remedies have been exhausted; it means 180 days after the discriminatory act *was committed.*

If your state or city has an FEP, the charges are passed to the state or local agency, which must act within 60 days. The EEOC must also, within 10 days after the charge has been received, notify your employer that a complaint has been filed. If the state or local agency does not act within that time, the charges are passed back to the EEOC, which has 120 days to investigate your charges, attempt to secure a conciliation agreement or bring a civil action in federal court (which is highly unlikely) against the employer or institute that has allegedly discriminated against you. In actual practice, the procedure may take years.

The key factor in any case is to determine as soon as possible what the procedure of your individual state is. Different states have different procedures, and it is important to learn what the process of your particular state is, whether you are covered and what time limits are involved.

In some states you may have to go to the agency office and fill out a special form with a counselor or caseworker, who will ask you questions about your complaint. In other states, you may be able to file a charge over the telephone or by mail. In many states, going through the agency is a prerequisite for any type of court action you may want to take in the event that you receive no satisfaction from the governing agency.

If you do not receive satisfaction from the state agency or if your case is dismissed, you may want to go to court on your own, and in this case you will probably have to obtain the services of a lawyer.

● *Phrasing your charge.* After you have determined the process for filing a charge and you have decided you want to file, you must make a written statement about the discriminatory activity that you want reconciled.

Draft your statement several times and read it over before filling in the complaint form. It is important that you phrase your complaint in a way that presents your case as strongly as possible. The burden is on you. If the agency believes you have a case within the boundaries of the law it will try to get your employer to stop discriminating—and this is why the initial statement is so important. State your facts clearly, keeping in mind that the major factor the person handling your case will look for is whether pregnancy has been treated equally with other physical conditions. It requires a certain mind set to look for this. Many people (and caseworkers are not different than others) do not have this mind set, so it is important to state your facts in such a way that your charge will not be turned down by the first person who sees your complaint.

The state will then review your case and determine whether or not the complaint is "actionable." If not, your case will be dismissed.

● *Following the investigation.* If the agency accepts your complaint, they will make an investigation that may or may not be thorough. It may take days or years.

The obvious question in this instance is whether or not you should bug the agency. It is always a good idea when dealing with a bureaucracy to keep in touch. Find out the name of the person handling your case. Let them know you are alive and interested, because they usually have a large case load and it's typical to keep the one that's uppermost in your mind on top of the file. The more informed and persistent you are, the more likely the agency will be to move along your case.

If the agency feels there is "reasonable cause" to believe that you have been discriminated against, they will try to conciliate your complaint with your employer. If the agency cannot reconcile your case, it will then issue a "notice of right to sue," which means you may then sue the discriminating party. The EEOC may decide to file a suit in federal court on your behalf. Keep in mind that this is highly unlikely, since the EEOC now has a policy of going after only "pattern and practice" cases, situations of large-scale discriminatory practices rather than individual ones.

If you do decide to sue, however, Title VII does provide that the courts appoint an attorney for you and that the fees be paid out of the settlement costs of the legal suit.

If the agency decides after its investigation that there has been no discrimination, then your case will be dismissed. At this point you may still want to go to court on your own. If you win, the court may stop your employer from discriminatory behavior, and order an affirmative action program, reinstatement of employees and back pay to be given to reinstated employees.

It's a lot of work, the process is usually frustrating and discouraging, and it can go on a long time. You may be angry initially and then simmer down, only to find you have a long wait for your case to make it through the bureaucracy. You may be the victim of retaliation or harassment (in which case, file another charge with the EEOC for retaliation, and sue for damages), and you may ultimately lose your job.

But—if you win, you may rectify an unfair practice and perhaps change the long-established discriminatory policies for those who follow you.

Filing a Complaint Through Your Union

Women who are members of unions have a unique opportunity to press for their rights by using the union structure to push for change. The collective-bargaining procedure can be effective in protecting women, because it gives the union power to negotiate contracts regarding aspects of the employer-employee relationship.

Although on the surface it may sound easy, the industry in which you work, its history and makeup, and the leadership of your union may all affect how you proceed in filing a complaint if you have reason to believe you have been discriminated against on the basis of pregnancy.

Before you do anything, learn as much as you can

about your union. Most unions are political, so it is important to know how yours works. Unions vary from those managed by professionally hired administrators to those run on a feudal system, with underlings swearing fealty to the chief. Learn how yours works. How are its leaders chosen? How are key decisions made? How does the collective-bargaining process work? Even if you have a progressive union leadership, the local may not be progressive.

Most unions, even those with large female memberships, are led by men, and for the most part sex discrimination and certainly pregnancy discrimination have not been considered priority issues. Union women often face a good deal of resistance from their male colleagues, and this resistance is hard to deal with. Few women have undertaken leadership roles in unions. There are few role models, little knowledge of how to act in a union business meeting and even less of the negotiating procedure.

Issues that unions tend to push for are economic ones. Fairer treatment and benefits for women mean less attention to men, and union leaders may not want to fight for the pregnancy rights of ten women at the expense of other issues involving two hundred men.

Unions view women with great suspicion. They're seen as marginal participants in the labor force and marginal members of the union. From a union standpoint, this may be a justifiable concern, because the men who stay in the union, who comprise its rank and file, have been there for twenty or twenty-five years and form a great power base. Women simply are not part of this.

Discreetly ask around *before* you approach the grievance committee to find out if similar types of grievances have been filed previously and how management has responded. Try to determine whether women are new to your union. How receptive is the union to women? Has this issue come up before? Have any other women-related issues come up, and how have they been handled? Does your union have any women officers or shop stewards? Are they sympathetic to the members—or loyal to the union leadership? If your union is comprised largely of male members, your grievance probably won't be taken as seriously as it would in a union with a larger percentage of female members.

Keep this in mind: Unions probably will not take the initiative; you will have to push for your rights.

Ideally, you should push for the inclusion of your pregnancy-based rights in your collective-bargaining agreements. It is most likely, however, that you will attempt to settle your complaint through the grievance procedure that is specified under the terms of your union contract. In most union contracts, the grievance procedure is good for only certain violations. If your particular situation is not covered, the grievance procedure may not be applicable. However, oftentimes business agents or shop stewards will take up individual problems with an employer and attempt to reconcile the complaint outside of the written contractual procedure.

Even if you are aware of the grievance procedure, it may be necessary to consider a little strategy because of the nature of the complaint. Know the proper procedure before filing a written complaint. Draft your complaint several times before actually filing out the grievance form. It is essential to state your case as strongly as possible without altering the facts.

Make sure your complaint is well documented. State that "so-and-so was present and said or did the following. So-and-so was also present and heard the following remarks."

It is absolutely essential to follow verbatim your contract in processing a grievance. There may be a time limit in filing one. Make sure you have read your contract thoroughly, know the proper procedure in your individual union for processing the complaint and know how a grievance is handled *according to your particular contract*.

Plan the strategy you will use to get the business agent or shop steward to support you. It is essential that you have the support of your shop steward or business agent in processing your complaint, and it is up to the individual woman to make sure this representative understands the nature and seriousness of the complaint. Many business agents are men, and in many instances, especially if women are relatively new to the union, they don't understand women on the job, are suspicious of them and may not want them in the union in the first place.

Pregnancy is not a debilitating illness—but you must make sure that your business agent knows this. He must feel certain that you are not going to use the union for improper purposes, but that you have a legitimate complaint and feel that you are the subject of discrimination.

It would not hurt—if your business agent seems reluctant to take you and your complaint seriously—to let your representative know that you are aware of your individual rights, that you know that if the union will not take action and you have a legitimate complaint, the union may be subject to an unfair-labor-practice claim, because it has not properly represented its member.

Your representative is apt to have more respect for a woman who also knows the proper combination of letters—for instance, OSHA (Occupational Safety and Health Administration), FEP (Fair Employment Practice) and EEOC (Equal Employment Opportunity Commission). Your representative may be apt to think, "Oh oh, I better watch out for this one. She knows her rights and maybe I better follow up on her claim."

If you still do not receive action, if there is still no support from the union business agent and you feel that you have gotten simply lip service toward your grievance, then send a letter to your business agent stating this, and indicate that if you do not receive action you may think of filing an unfair-labor-practice suit against the union.

At this point, the union representative may call his legal counsel and ask what to do. The lawyer will most likely tell him to do his job and process the claim for two reasons: (1) If the employee does have a legitimate complaint, then it should be resolved. The union will have a good record in representing its membership, and this will help in recruiting future members. (2) If a woman does file an unfair labor practice against the union, then the union will have documentation that it did in fact process the claim properly.

If the claim has not been processed properly within the union grievance machinery, then file a claim with a state or federal agency. (See pages 245–49.)

Unions are concerned with criticism. They have been the spotlight of numerous legislative hearings, and they don't want to get involved in excessive administrative decisions. The fact that someone files a complaint in a union situation is a presumption of guilt; there is tremendous pressure to settle the complaint, not necessarily because of the rightness of the charge, but, rather, for the union to save its own neck and avoid any negative publicity.

In addition, there is a strong interrelationship of discrimination laws. Chances are that if there is suspicion of pregnancy-based discrimination, there will also be suspicion of sex discrimination.

If you file a complaint with an outside agency and you win, there is a chance that the union will be charged for not representing you properly. The union wants to avoid this at all costs.

So stand your ground, talk to the other women in your union who are in similar situations, talk to women in other unions, organize women's caucuses and raise issues that are women's issues, specifically within the context of contract negotiations. As one female labor leader explained: "That's a completely different thing than saying to the male leadership, 'We'd like you to raise these issues for us.'"

Resources for Legal Assistance: State Agencies Usually Handling Labor or Employment Matters

Alabama

Department of Industrial Relations
Industrial Relations Bldg.
Montgomery 36104

Alabama Department of Labor
State Administrative Bldg.
Suite 600
Montgomery 36104
(Administrators labor-relations law, and occupational safety and health act)

Alaska

Alaska Department of Labor
P.O. Box 1149
Juneau 99801

Alaska State Commission for Human Rights
5th Fl., MacKay Bldg.
338 Denali St.
Anchorage 99501

Arizona

Industrial Commission
1601 West Jefferson St.
P.O. Box 19070
Phoenix 85005

Employment Security Commission
1717 West Jefferson St.
P.O. Box 6123
Phoenix 85005

Arizona Civil Rights Commission
1502 West Jefferson St.
Phoenix 85007

Arkansas

Department of Labor
Capitol Hill Bldg.
Little Rock 72201

California

Fair Employment Practices Commission
455 Golden Gate Ave.
P.O. Box 603
San Francisco 94101

Department of Industrial Relations
State Building Annex
455 Golden Gate Ave.
San Francisco 94102

Department of Human Resources Development
800 Capitol Mall
Sacramento 95814

Colorado

Department of Labor
and Employment
200 East Ninth Ave.
Denver 80203

Colorado Civil Rights
Commission
Rm. 312, State Services
Bldg.
1525 Sherman St.
Denver 80203

Connecticut

Labor Department
200 Folly Brook Blvd.
Hartford 06115

Commission on Human
Rights and Opportunities
90 Washington St.
Hartford 06115

Delaware

Department of Labor
801 West St.
Wilmington 19899

Division of Industrial
Affairs
Department of Labor
618 No. Union St.
Wilmington 19805

District of Columbia

D.C. Commission on
Human Relations
District Bldg., Rm. 22
14th & E Sts., N.W.
Washington, D.C. 20004

Florida

Department of
Commerce
Collins Bldg.
Tallahassee 32304

Georgia

Department of Labor
State Labor Bldg.
Atlanta 30334

Hawaii

Department of Labor and
Industrial Relations
825 Mililani St.
Honolulu 96813

Idaho

Commission on Human
Rights
Department of Social
Services
Statehouse
Boise 83702

Department of Labor
317 Main St.
P.O. Box 7189
Boise 83707

Illinois

Fair Employment
Practices Commission
160 N. LaSalle St.
Chicago 60601

Department of Labor
160 N. LaSalle St.
Chicago 60601

Industrial Commission
160 N. LaSalle St.
Chicago 60601

Fair Employment
Practices Commission
9th Fl., 189 West
Madison St.
Chicago 60602

Indiana

Division of Labor
Indiana State Office
Bldg.,
Rm. 1013
100 N. Senate Ave.
Indianapolis 46204

Civil Rights Commission
410 State Office Bldg.
100 N. Senate Ave.
Indianapolis 46204

Iowa

Bureau of Labor
State House
East 7th and Court Ave.
4th Fl.
Des Moines 50319

Iowa Civil Rights
Commission
State Capitol Bldg.
Des Moines 50319

Kansas

Department of Labor
401 Topeka Ave.
Topeka 66603

Commission on Civil
Rights
State Office Bldg.
Topeka 66612

Kentucky

Department of Labor
State Office Bldg. Annex
Frankfort 40601

Commission on Human
Rights
26 Capitol Annex Bldg.
Frankfort 40601

Louisiana

Department of Labor
205 Capitol Annex
P.O. Box 44063
Baton Rouge 70804

Maine

Department of Labor and
Industry
State Office Bldg.
Augusta 04330

Maine Human Rights
Commission
Augusta 04330

Maryland

State of Maryland
Commission on Human
Relations
Mount Vernon Bldg.
701 St. Paul St.
Baltimore 21202

Massachusetts

Department of Labor
and Industries
State Office Bldg.
Government Center
100 Cambridge St.
Boston 02202

Commission Against
Discrimination
296 Boylston St.
Boston 02108

Michigan

Department of Labor
300 E. Michigan Ave.
Lansing 48913

Civil Rights Commission
1000 Cadillac Square
Bldg.
Detroit 48226

Minnesota

Department of Human
Rights
60 State Office Bldg.
St. Paul 55155

Mississippi

Employment Security
Commission
P.O. Box 1699
Jackson 39205

Missouri

Missouri Department of
Labor and Industrial
Relations
1904 Missouri Blvd.
Jefferson City 65101

Missouri Commission on
Human Rights
314 E. High, Box 1129
Jefferson City 65101

Montana

Department of Labor and
Industry
1331 Helena Ave.
Helena 59601

Nebraska

Nebraska Equal
Opportunity Commission
233 South 14th St.
Lincoln 68509

Nevada

Nevada Department of
Labor
111 W. Telegraph St.
Rm. 214
Carson City 89701

Nevada Commission on
Equal Rights of Citizens
215 East Bonanza Rd.
Las Vegas 89101

New Hampshire

Department of Labor
1 Pillsbury St.
Concord 03301

New Hampshire
Commission for Human
Rights
166 South St.
Concord 03301

New Jersey

Department of Labor
and Industry
Labor and Industry
Bldg.
John Fitch Plaza
Trenton 08625

New Jersey Public
Employment Relations
Commission
New Jersey Labor and
Industry Bldg.
P.O. Box V
Trenton 08625

New Mexico

Labor and Industrial
Commission
137 E. DeVargas St.
Santa Fe 87501

Human Rights
Commission
Villagra Bldg., Rm. 121
408 Galisteo St.
Santa Fe 87501

New York

Department of Labor
State Campus
Albany 12226

Division of Human Rights
270 Broadway
New York City 10007

North Carolina

Department of Labor
P.O. Box 1151
Raleigh 27602

North Dakota

Department of Labor
State Capitol
Bismarck 58501

Ohio

Civil Rights Commission
240 Parsons Ave.
Columbus 43215

Oklahoma

Department of Labor
State Capitol
Oklahoma City 73105

Human Rights
Commission
P.O. Box 52945
Oklahoma City 73102

Oregon

Bureau of Labor
115 Labor and
Industries Bldg.
Salem 97310

Civil Rights Division
Bureau of Labor
State Office Bldg., Rm.
466
Portland 97201

Pennsylvania

Department of Labor and
Industry
Labor and Industry Bldg.
Harrisburg 17120

Pennsylvania Human
Relations Commission
100 North Cameron St.
Harrisburg 17101

Rhode Island

Department of Labor
235 Promenade St.
Providence 02908

Commission for Human
Rights
244 Broad St.
Providence 02903

South Carolina

Department of Labor
1710 Gervais St.
P.O. Box 11329
Columbia 29211

South Dakota

Department of Labor and
Management Relations
State Capitol Bldg.
Pierre 57501

Commission on Human
Relations
5th and Highland
Sioux Falls 57103

Tennessee

Department of Labor
C1-100 Cordell Hull Bldg.
Nashville 37219

Texas

Bureau of Labor
Statistics
Box 12157, Capitol Sta.
Austin 78711

Utah

Industrial Commission
State Capitol Bldg.
Salt Lake City 84114

Vermont

Department of Labor and
Industry
State Office Bldg.
Montpelier 05602

Virginia

Department of Labor
and Industry
P.O. Box 1814
Ninth Street Office Bldg.
Richmond 23214

Washington

Washington State
Human Rights Commission
1411 Fourth Avenue
Bldg.
Seattle 98101

West Virginia

Department of Labor
Capitol Complex
1900 Washington St.,
East
Charleston 25305

State Human Rights
Commission
1591 East Washington St.
Charleston 25305

Wisconsin

Equal Rights Division
Department of Industry,
Labor and Human
Relations
201 E. Washington Ave.
Madison 53703

Wyoming

Department of Labor and
Statistics
304 Capitol Bldg.
Cheyenne 82001

Fair Employment
Practices Commission
304 Capitol Bldg.
Cheyenne 82001

Puerto Rico

Department of Labor
414 Barbosa Ave.
Hato Rey 00917

Offices of the Equal Employment Opportunity Commission

The following is a list of federal district offices of the Equal Employment Opportunity Commission. Call or write for information regarding filing a charge about any presumed discriminatory pattern or practice.

Albuquerque Area Office
Western Bank Bldg.
Suite 115
505 Marquette Ave.,
N.W.
Albuquerque, N. Mex.
87101
505 766-2016

Atlanta District Office
Citizens Trust Bldg.,
10th Fl.
75 Piedmont Ave., N.E.
Atlanta, Ga. 30303
404 221-4566

Baltimore District Office
Rotunda Bldg., Suite
210
711 W. 40th St.
Baltimore, Md. 21211
301 962-3932

Birmingham District Office
2121 8th Ave., N.
Birmingham, Ala. 35203
205 254-1166

Boston Area Office
150 Causeway St., Suite
1000
Boston, Mass. 02114
617 223-4535

Buffalo Area Office
One W. Genesse St., Rm.
320
Buffalo, N.Y. 14202
716 846-4441

Charlotte District Office
1301 Morehead St.
Charlotte, N.C. 28204
704 371-6137

Chicago District Office
Federal Bldg., Rm. 234
536 S. Clark St.
Chicago, Ill. 60605
312 353-2713

Cincinnati Area Office
Federal Bldg., Rm. 7015
550 Main St.
Cincinnati, Ohio 45202
513 684-2379

Cleveland District Office
Engineers' Bldg., Rm.
602
1365 Ontario St.
Cleveland, Ohio 44114
216 522-7425

Dallas District Office
1900 Pacific—13th Fl.
Dallas, Tex. 75201
214 767-4607

Dayton Area Office
Federal Bldg.
200 W. Second St.
Dayton, Ohio 45402
513 225-2753

Denver District Office
1513 Stout St., 6th Fl.
Denver, Colo, 80202
303 837-2771

Detroit District Office
660 Woodward Ave.
Suite 600
Detroit, Mich. 48226
313 226-7636

El Paso Area Office
Property Trust Bldg.
2211 E. Missouri, Rm.
E-235
El Paso, Tex. 79903
915 543-7596

Fresno Area Office
1303 P. St.
Suite 103
Fresno, Calif. 93721
209 487-5703

Greensboro Area Office
324 W. Market St.
Rm. 132
Greensboro, S.C. 27402
919 378-5174

Greenville Area Office
Bankers Trust Bldg., 5th
Fl.
7 N. Laurens St.
Greenville, S.C. 29601
803 233-1791

Houston District Office
Federal Bldg., Rm. 1101
2320 LaBranch
Houston, Tex. 77004
713 226-5611

Indianapolis District
Office
Federal Bldg.
U.S. Courthouse
46 E. Ohio St., Rm. 456
Indianapolis, Ind. 46204
317 269-7212

Jackson Area Office
100 W. Capitol St.
Suite 721
Jackson, Miss. 39201
601 969-4537

Kansas City Area Office
1150 Grand Ave., 1st Fl.
Kansas City, Mo. 64106
816 374-5773

Little Rock Area Office
Federal Bldg.
700 W. Capitol St.
Little Rock, Ark. 72201
501 378-5901

Los Angeles District Office
3255 Wilshire Blvd., 9th
Fl.
Los Angeles, Calif.
90010
213 798-3400

Louisville Area Office
U.S. Post Office &
Courthouse
600 Jefferson St.
Louisville, Ky. 40202
502 582-6082

Memphis District Office
1407 Union Ave., Suite
502
Memphis, Tenn. 38104
901 521-2617

Miami District Office
DuPont Plaza Center
Suite 414
300 Biscayne Blvd. Way
Miami, Fla. 33131
305 350-4491

Milwaukee District
Office
342 N. Water St., Rm.
612
Milwaukee, Wis. 53202
414 291-1111

Minneapolis Area Office
Plymouth Bldg.
12 S. Sixth St.
Minneapolis, Minn. 55402
612 725-6101

Nashville Area Office
Parkway Towers
404 James Robertson Pky.
Nashville, Tenn. 37219
615 251-5820

Newark Area Office
744 Broad St., Suite 502
Newark, N.J. 07102
201 645-6383

New Orleans District
Office
F. Edward Hébert
Federal Bldg.
600 South St.
New Orleans, La. 70130
504 589-3842

New York District Office
90 Church St.
Rm. 1301
New York, N.Y. 10007
212 264-7161

Norfolk Area Office
200 Granby Mall
Rm. 412
Norfolk, Va. 23510
804 441-3470

Oakland Area Office
George P. Miller
Federal Bldg.
1515 Clay St., Rm. 640
Oakland, Calif. 94612
415 273-7588

Oklahoma City Area
Office
50 Penn Pl., Suite 1430
Oklahoma City, Okla.
73118
405 231-4912

Philadelphia District Office
127 N. Fourth St., Suite
300
Philadelphia, Pa. 19106
216 597-7784

Phoenix District Office
201 N. Central Ave.
Suite 1450
Phoenix, Ariz. 85073
602 261-3882

Pittsburgh Area Office
Federal Bldg., Rm.
2038A
1000 Liberty Ave.
Pittsburgh, Pa. 15222
412 644-3444

Raleigh Area Office
414 Fayetteville St.
Raleigh, N.C. 27608
919 755-4064

Richmond Area Office
400 N. Eighth St., Rm.
6213
Richmond, Va. 23219
804 782-2911

San Antonio Area Office
727 E. Durango, Suite
B-601
San Antonio, Tex. 78206
512 229-6051

San Diego Area Office
San Diego Federal Bldg.
880 Front St.
San Diego, Calif. 92188
714 556-0260

San Francisco District
Office
1390 Market St., Suite
325
San Francisco, Calif.
94102
415 556-0260

San Jose Area Office
Crocker Plaza Bldg.
84 W. Santa Clara, Rm.
300
San Jose, Calif. 95113
408 275-7352

Seattle District Office
Dexter Horton Bldg.
710 Second Ave.
Seattle, Wash. 98104
206 422-0976

St. Louis District Office
1601 Olive St.
St. Louis, Mo. 63103
314 425-5571

Tampa Area Office
700 Twiggs St., Rm. 302
Tampa, Fla. 33602
813 228-2310

Washington, D.C., Area
Office
1717 H St., N.W., Suite
402
Washington, D.C. 20006
202 653-6197

NOTES

CHAPTER 1
AT WORK

Because this chapter includes material on both work and legal issues, we have divided our references accordingly. We hope this will enable our readers to pursue specific areas of interest with greater ease.

Development of this chapter included interviews with pregnant women in a variety of fields and at different levels of achievement. Participants were recruited through author's queries placed in a series of professional publications, including the following professional associations: the National Education Association, the American Bar Association, the American Sociological Association, the Union Women's Alliance to Gain Equality, Federally Employed Women, the National Association of Physician Nurses, the American Association of School Librarians, the National League for Nursing and the National Extension Homemaker's Council. An advertisement was also placed in *MBA Communications*.

Interviews were conducted with approximately one hundred executives responsible for public or employee relations, who were arbitrarily selected from companies listed in the *Fortune* magazine directory of the five hundred largest U.S. industrial concerns.

For those areas dealing with work, in addition to those

people mentioned in the text or in the references below, interviews were conducted with Janet Giele, professor of sociology, Brandeis University, Waltham, Massachusetts, and author of *Women and the Future;* Judith M. Bardwick, associate dean and professor of psychology, University of Michigan, Ann Arbor, Michigan, and author of *In Transition: How Feminism, Sexual Liberation, and the Search for Self-fulfillment Have Altered Our Lives;* Kristin Moore, research associate, The Urban Institute, Washington, D.C.; Debby King, research assistant, Hospital and Health Care Employees, The Urban Institute, Washington, D.C.; and Dr. Samuel Epstein, professor of public health, University of Illinois Medical School, Chicago, Illinois.

Interviews regarding legal issues were conducted with Eleanor Holmes Norton, chair, Equal Employment Opportunity Commission; Ruth Weyand, supervisory trial attorney, EEOC; Kerry Nicholas, staff attorney, Women's Law Project, Philadelphia; Carol Schiro Greenwald, research associate, Institute for Independent Study, Radcliffe College; Ira Drogin, Leaf, Kurzman, Duell and Drogin, New York City; Susan Ross, visiting professor of law, George Washington University, Washington, D.C.; and Ann Thatcher Anderson, general counsel, New York State Civil Rights Commission.

Work-Related Issues

GENERAL REFERENCES

Jessie Bernard, *The Future of Motherhood* (New York: The Dial Press, 1974).

William H. Chafe, *The American Woman: Her Changing Social, Economic and Political Roles, 1920–1970* (New York: Oxford University Press, 1972).

William H. Chafe, *Women and Equality: Changing Patterns in American Culture* (New York: Oxford University Press, 1977).

Jane R. Chapman, ed., "Economic Independence for Women: The Foundation for Equal Rights," *Sage Yearbook in Women's Policy Studies,* vol. 1. (Beverly Hills, Calif.: Sage Publications, 1976).

Jane R. Chapman and Margaret Gates, eds., *Women Into Wives: The Legal and Economic Impact of Marriage* (Beverly Hills, Calif.: Sage Publications, 1977).

Cynthia Fuchs Epstein, *Women's Place: Options and Limits in Professional Careers* (Berkeley, Calif.: University of California Press, 1970).

Janet Giele, *Women and the Future* (New York: The Free Press, 1978).

Margaret Henning and Anne Jardim, *The Managerial Woman* (Garden City, N.Y.: Anchor Press, 1977).

Andrea Hricko with Melanie Brunt, *Working for Your Life: A Woman's Guide to Job-Health Hazards,* Joint publication of the Labor Occupational Health Program, the Center for Labor Research and Education, the Institute of Industrial Relations, University of California at Berkeley, and the Public Citizen's Health Research Group, Washington, D.C., 1976.

Huber Joan, ed., *Changing Women in a Changing Society* (Chicago: University of Chicago Press, 1973).

Vilma Hunt, "Occupational Health Problems of Pregnant Women: A Report and Recommendations for the Office of the Secretary," Department of HEW, April 1975.

Rosabeth Moss Kantor, *Men and Women of the Corporation* (New York: Basic Books, 1977).

Juanita M. Kreps, ed., "Women and the American Economy: A Look to the 1980s," The American Assembly, Columbia University, 1976.

Letty Cottin Pogrebin, *Getting Yours* (New York: David McKay, 1975).

Catherine Samuels, *The Forgotten Five Million: Women in Public Employment* (New York: Women's Action Alliance, 1975).

Jeanne M. Stellman and Susan Daum, *Work is Dangerous to Your Health* (New York: Vintage Books, 1973).

Jeanne M. Stellman, *Women's Work, Women's Health: Myths and Realities* (New York: Pantheon Books, 1977).

Work-Related Journals, Periodicals and Documents

Larry L. Bumpers and James. A. Sweet, "Patterns of Employment Before and After Childbirth," CDE Working Paper 77–20, Center for Demography and Ecology, University of Wisconsin.

The American College of Obstetricians and Gynecologists, *Guidelines on Pregnancy and Work* (ACOG: Chicago, 1977).

ACOG Technical Bulletin, Number 58–May 1980, "Pregnancy, Work and Disability."

Gerry E. Hendershot, "Work During Pregnancy and Subsequent Hospitalization of Mothers and Infants: Evidence from the National Survey of Family Growth," Paper prepared for presentation to the annual meeting of the Population Association of America, Atlanta, April 14, 1978.

Rosabeth Moss Kantor, "Work in a New America," *Daedalus,* 107:1, Winter 1978, pp. 47–78.

Alice S. Rossi, "A Biosocial Perspective on Parenting," *Daedalus,* 106:2, Spring 1977, pp. 1–31.

Alice S. Rossi, "Equality Between the Sexes: An Immodest Proposal," *Daedalus,* 93:2, Spring 1964, pp. 607–52.

Ralph E. Smith, *Prospects for Women in the Paid Labor Market,* The Urban Institute, Washington, D.C., June 1978.

"Men and Women" series, The New York *Times,* Nov. 27, 28, 29 and 30, 1977.

"Working in Pregnancy: How Long? How Hard? What's Your Role?" Symposium: Contemporary OB/GYN, September 1980, vol. 16, no. 3

"Women at Work" Series, *The Wall Street Journal,* Aug. 28, 31; Sept. 5, 8, 13, 15, 19 and 22, 1978.

U.S. Department of Labor, Women's Bureau, *1975 Handbook on Women Workers,* Bulletin 297, Washington, D.C., 1975.

Legal References

SUPREME COURT DECISIONS

Phillips v. *Martin Marietta Corp.*, 400 U.S. 542 (1971).

Griggs v. *Duke Power Co.*, 401 U.S. 424 (1971).

Cleveland Board of Education v. *LaFleur*, 414 U.S. 632 (1974).

Geduldig v. *Aiello*, 417 U.S. 484 (1974).

General Electric Co. v. *Gilbert*, 429 U.S. 125 (1976).

Nashville Gas Co. v. *Satty*, 46 USLW 4026, Dec. 6, 1977.

Books Regarding Legal Issues

Barbara A. Brown, Ann E. Freedman, Harriet N. Katz, and Alice M. Price, *Women's Rights and the Law* (New York: Praeger Publishers, 1977).

U.S. House of Representatives, Subcommittee on Employment Opportunities, *Hearings: Legislation to Prohibit Sex Discrimination on the Basis of Pregnancy*, 95 Cong., 1 sess., April 7, 1977.

Vilma Hunt, "Occupational Health Problems of Pregnant Women," Report and recommendations for the Office of the Secretary, HEW, April 1975.

Susan Deller Ross, *The Rights of Women* (New York: Avon Books, 1973).

Catherine Samuels, *The Forgotten Five Million: Women in Public Employment* (New York: Women's Action Alliance, 1975).

Jeanne Stellman and Susan Daum, *Work is Dangerous to Your Health* (New York: Vintage Books, 1973).

Jeanne M. Stellman, *Women's Work, Women's Health: Myths and Realities* (New York: Pantheon Books, 1977).

U.S. Senate, Subcommittee on Labor of the Committee on Human Resources, *Hearings: Discrimination on the*

Basis of Pregnancy, 1977, 95 Cong., 1 sess., S. 995, April 26, 27 and 29, 1977.

Periodicals and Documents—Legal Issues

"A Pregnancy Ruling That Could Cost $1.6 Billion," *Business Week,* Nov. 29, 1976, p. 41.

"The Dilemma of Regulating Reproductive Risks," *Business Week,* Aug. 29, 1977, pp. 76–82.

Thomas J. Gillooley, Edwin T. Holmes and John R. Hurley, "The Irrational Trend Toward Mandatory Maternity Coverage," *Drake Law Review,* vol. 26:4, 1977.

Ruth Bader Ginsburg and Susan Deller Ross, "Pregnancy and Discrimination," *The New York Times,* Jan. 25, 1977, p. 35.

Carol Schiro Greenwald, "Women's Rights, Courts and Congress: Conflict Over Pregnancy Disability Compensation Policies," Paper prepared for delivery at the annual meeting, American Political Science Association, New York, Sept. 3, 1978.

Linda H. Kistler and Carol C. McDonough, "Paid Maternity Leave—Benefits May Justify the Cost," *Labor Law Journal,* Dec. 1975, pp. 782–94.

"Pregnant Decisions," *Newsweek,* Dec. 20, 1976, p. 59.

"Senate Votes Pregnancy Benefits in Disability Plans for Workers," *The New York Times,* Sept. 17, 1977, p. 8.

"Justices, 9–0, Block a Loss of Seniority in Maternity Leave," *The New York Times,* Dec. 7, 1977, p. 1.

Letty Cottin Pogrebin, "Anatomy Isn't Destiny," *The New York Times,* May 6, 1977, p. 29.

Katherine Stone, *Handbook for OCAW Women,* Oil, Chemical and Atomic Workers International Union, Denver, 1973.

"No Pay for Pregnancy," *Time,* Dec. 20, 1976, p. 72.

Title VII, *Civil Rights Act of 1964,* as amended (78 Stat. 253, 86 Stat. 103, 42 USC s20000e, *et seq.*).

"Agencies Discourage Exclusion of Women from Hazardous Jobs (OSHA–EEOC), Companies Warned Their Policies May Be Discriminatory," *The Regulatory Alert,* Research Institute of America, May 24, 1978.

Ruth Weyand, Equal Opportunity Employment Conference, New Orleans, Nov. 1977, "Pregnancy-Related Disabilities—Impact of Supreme Court Decisions; New Directions and Legislation."

Work-Related Particular References
Publications

"The Future of the American Family," Testimony of Paul C. Glick, senior demographer, U.S. Department of Commerce, Bureau of the Census, before the Select Committee on Population, U.S. House of Representatives, May 23, 1978.

Judith Blake, "Coercive Pronatalism and American Population Policy," reprint 434, International Population and Urban Research, Institute of International Studies, University of California at Berkeley. Originally prepared for the commission on Population Growth and The American Future: Research Reports, vol. VI, *Aspects of Population Growth Policy,* ed. Robert Parke, Jr., and Charles F. Westoff.

U.S. Working Women: A Databook, U.S. Department of Labor bulletin, Bureau of Labor Statistics, 1977.

Interviews

Dr. Samuel Epstein, professor of public health, University of Illinois Medical School, Chicago; Andrea Hricko, labor coordinator, Labor Occupational Health Program, Center for Labor Research and Education, Institute of Industrial Relations, University of California at Berkeley.

Proceedings

Eula Bingham, Ph.D., ed., *Conference on Women and the Workplace,* Society for Occupational and Environmental Health, Washington, D.C., 1977.

CHAPTER 2
TAKING CHARGE OF YOUR MEDICAL CARE

Preparation of this chapter included attendance at the 1978 annual clinical meeting of the American College of Obstetricians and Gynecologists, Anaheim, California, April 1978; "The Birth of an American Child," a conference sponsored by the National Institute for the Psychotherapies, including a panel discussion of "The Psychology of Alternative Methods of Childbirth." Also reflected in the chapter is an interview with Dr. Martin Stone, 1978 President-Elect of ACOG.

General References

Jack A. Pritchard and Paul C. Macdonald, *Williams Obstetrics,* 15th ed. (New York: Appleton-Century-Crofts, 1976).

Ralph Benson and associate authors, *Current Obstetric and Gynecologic Diagnosis and Treatment* (Los Altos, Calif.: Lange Medical Publications, 1976).

Seymour L. Romney, M.D., Mary Jane Gray, M.D., A. Brian Little, M.D., James A. Merrill, M.D., E. J. Quilligan, M.D., and Richard Stander, M.D., *Gynecology and Obstetrics: The Health Care of Women* (New York: McGraw-Hill, 1975).

Roy M. Pitkin, M.D., ed., *The Year Book of Obstetrics and Gynecology,* former ed. J. P. Greenhill, Year Book Medical Publishers, 1970–78.

ACOG, *Précis: An Update in Obstetrics and Gynecology* (New York: McGraw-Hill, 1977).

National Center for Health Services Research, *Women and Their Health: Research Implications for a New Era,* ed. Virginia Olesen, Ph.D., U.S. Department of Health, Education and Welfare, HRA 77–3138.

Survey of selected women's magazines from 1910–78.

Survey of *Ob-Gyn News,* published by the International Medical News Group, Rockville, Maryland.

Surveys of publications of ACOG; March of Dimes Birth Defects Foundation; International Childbirth Education Association; Boston Women's Health Book Collective; U.S. Department Maternal Child Health.

Particular References

McCall's magazine, vol. 8, Dec. 1952, p. 38.

ACOG, *Standards for Obstetric-Gynecologic Services,* 1974.

Richard W. Wertz and Dorothy C. Wertz, *Lying-In: A History of Childbirth in America* (New York: The Free Press, 1977).

ICEA, *1978 Biennial Report,* pp. 4–5.

Marjorie Karmel, *Thank You, Dr. Lamaze* (New York: Dolphin Books, 1965).

Richard Aubry, M.D., *What Is 'Family-Centered' Obstetrics?* Ortho Panel 29, Science and Medicine Publishing, 1978, p. 14.

ACOG and the American Academy of Family Physicians, "Core Curriculum and Hospital Practice Privileges in Obstetrics and Gynecology for Family Physicians," statement of policy.

HMO, *Medical World News,* March 6, 1978, p. 76.

ACOG/NACOG, statement on mutual relationship, 1974; NACOG, *Nursing Standards Functions and Standards,* 1974.

American College of Nurse-Midwives information is from the following sources: Barbara Brennan and Joan Rattner Heilman, *The Complete Book of Midwifery* (New York: E.P. Dutton, 1977); T. Schely Gatewood, M.D., and Richard B. Stewart, M.D., "Obstetricians and Nurse-Midwives: The Team Approach in Private Practice," *American Journal of Obstetrics and Gynecology,* vol. 123:1, Sept. 1, 1975, pp. 35–40.

"An Assessment of the Hazards of Amniocentesis: Report to the Medical Research Council," *British Journal of Obstetrics and Gynecology,* suppl. 2, vol. 85, 1978.

March of Dimes Birth Defects Foundation, *Genetic Counselling*.

March of Dimes Birth Defects Foundation, *Toward Improving the Outcome of Pregnancy: Recommendations for the Regional Development of Maternal and Perinatal Health Services*.

Department of Health, Education and Welfare, Health Resource Administration, *National Guidelines for Health Planning*, pp. 51–54.

"Consumers Call for Changes," *ICEA News*, vol. 16, Winter 1977–78, p. 1.

Commentary on National Guidelines for Health Planning (New York: The Maternity Center, Dec. 1977); Ruth Watson Lubic, R.N., M.A., C.M.M.; "Comprehensive Maternity Care as an Ambulatory Service–Maternity Center Association's Birth Alternative," *Journal of the New York State Nurses Association*, vol. 8:4, Dec. 1977.

"Hospitals Bow to Couples Wanting Special Births," *Medical World News*, Oct. 3, 1977, p. 38.

"Yale to Revoke Privileges for Home Birth," *Ob-Gyn News*, vol. 13:2, Jan. 15, 1978; "ACOG Official: Home Delivery 'Maternal Trauma, Child Abuse,' " *Ob-Gyn News*, vol. 12:19, p. 1.

"Higher Mortality Rate Found in Home Births," *ACOG Newsletter*, vol. 22:2, Feb. 1978.

Response to article quoting ACOG officials on dangers of home delivery: Dr. Lewis B. Mehl, M.D., of the Institute for Childbirth and Family Research, Chapel Hill, N.C., *Ob-Gyn News*, vol. 13:1, Jan. 1, 1978.

"It Would Be Premature to Say Home Delivery Isn't Safe," *Ob-Gyn News*, vol. 13:3, Feb. 1, 1978.

ACOG, *Standards for Ambulatory Obstetric Care*, 1974, pp. 3–7.

Barbara Yuncker, "Helping Nature Too Much is Unnatural and Dangerous," New York *Post*, Nov. 28, 1977, p. 33.

Suzanne Arms, *Immaculate Deception* (New York: Bantam Books, 1977).

Peter M. Dunn, "Obstetric Delivery Today—For Better or Worse?" Paper delivered at a scientific meeting of the Royal College of Obstetricians and Gynecologists, Feb. 4, 1976. Reprinted in *The Lancet*, April 10, 1976.

Discussion of an article on midwifery: Dr. Allan G. W. Mcleod, *American Journal of Obstetrics and Gynecology*, vol. 123:1, Sept. 1, 1975, p. 38.

"Modified Leboyer Delivery Proved So Physiologically Safe It Is Being Used Routinely," *Ob-Gyn News*, Oct. 15, 1977, pp. 1 and 34.

Doris Haire, "The Cultural Warping of Childbirth," *ICEA News*, Sept. 1972, p. 6.

"Fetal Heart Rate Monitoring," *ACOG Technical Bulletin*, 32, June 1975; Statement by Donald Kennedy, Food and Drug Administration commissioner, before Senate Subcommittee on Health and Scientific Research, April 17, 1978; Comments by witnesses reported in *Washington Drug and Device Letter*, April 24, 1978; Judith Randall, "Is Fetal Monitoring Safe? Widely Used Technique Needs More Testing," Washington *Post*, April 16, 1978; "Mother's View on Fetal Monitor May Affect Child Later," *Ob-Gyn News*, vol. 13:3, Feb. 1, 1978, p. 21.

"Malpractice Update: More Suits Against Ob-Gyns," *Contemporary Ob/Gyn*, vol. II, April 1978, p. 13; "Which Doctors Get Sued and Why," *Medical World News*, Dec. 1, 1975, p. 19; "Child Can Sue for Preconception Damages," *Medical World News*, Sept. 1, 1977, p. 16; "Malpractice: The Grim Outlook for '76," *Medical World News*, Dec. 12, 1976; Diana Copsey, "Fear of Suit Said to Drive Up Rate of Cesarian Sections," *Ob-Gyn News*, May 15, 1978, vol. 13:10, pp. 1 and 33.

"Few OB Complications Will Require C-Section," *Ob-Gyn News*, July 15, 1978.

Induction of Labor, ACOG Technical Bulletin 49, May 1978.

John S. Haller, "Abuses in Gynecology Surgery—An Historical Appraisal," *Women and Their Health*, pp. 27–33.

Gena Corea, *The Hidden Malpractice: How American Medicine Treats Women as Patients and Professionals* (New York: William Morrow, 1977).

Mary C. Howell, M.D., Ph.D., "What Medical Schools Teach About Women," *New England Journal of Medicine*, Aug. 8, 1974, pp. 304–7.

Kay Weiss, "What Medical Students Learn About Women," *Seizing Our Bodies: The Politics of Women's Health* (New York: Vintage Books, 1977).

Robert Mendenhall, M.S., Warren Pearse, M.D., Richard Stander, M.D., and Albert Isenman, M.B.A., "Manpower for Obstetrics and Gynecology: Demographic Considerations and Practice Work Load," *American Journal of Obstetrics and Gynecology*, April 15, 1978, pp. 927–932.

Charlotte Muller, "Methodological Issues in Health Economic Research Relevant to Women," *Women and Their Health*, p. 47.

CHAPTER 3
SPORTS

In addition to the persons cited in the text, background interviews were conducted with Marge Albohm, head trainer, Indiana University at Bloomington, and member, executive board, American Alliance for Health, Physical Education and Recreation; and Eve Auchincloss, executive director, Women's Sports Foundation, San Mateo, Calif.

General References

Dorothy V. Harris, "The Pregnant Athlete," *Womensports*, June 1977, p. 46.

Ekaterina Azharieva, M.D., "Olympic Participation by Women—Effects on Pregnancy and Childbirth," *JAMA*, vol. 221:9, Aug. 28, 1972, pp. 992–95.

Ellen Weber, "Three Great Myths of Sex and Sports," *Womensports,* pp. 30–33; 57–60.

Carol Dilfer, *Your Baby, Your Body* (New York: Crown Publishers, 1977).

"Roundtable: Sports During Pregnancy, Other Questions Explored," *The Physician and Sportsmedicine,* vol. 4, March 1976, pp. 82–85.

Howard G. Knuttgen and Kendall Emerson, Jr., "Physiological Response to Pregnancy at Rest and During Exercise," *Journal of Applied Physiology,* vol. 36:5, May 1974, pp. 549–53.

E.S. Gendel, "Pregnancy, Fitness and Sports," *JAMA,* vol. 201, pp. 751, 754.

Dr. Joan Ullyot, *Women's Running* (Mt. View, Calif.: World Publications, 1976), pp. 120–21.

Kathie Samuelson, "Schlepping Through Pregnancy," *The Jogger,* vol. 9, no. 49, Dec. 1977, pp. 7, 14.

Bob Glover and Jack Sheperd, *The Runner's Handbook* (New York: Viking, 1978).

Particular References

Gyula J. Erdelyi, "Gynecological Survey of Female Athletes," *Journal of Sports Medicine and Physical Fitness,* vol. 2, 1962, pp. 174–79.

"Roundtable: Pregnancy and Sports," *The Physician and Sportsmedicine,* May 1974, pp. 35–41.

Evalyn S. Gendel, M.D., "Lack of Fitness a Source of Chronic Ills in Women," *The Physician and Sportsmedicine,* vol. 6, no. 2, Feb. 1978, pp. 85–95.

Dr. Carl Javert, *Spontaneous and Habitual Abortion* (New York: McGraw-Hill, 1957).

C. T. Javert, "Further Follow-up on Habitual Abortion Patients," *American Journal of Obstetrics and Gynecology,* 84:1149, 1962.

Dr. Josephine H. Kenyon, "Waiting for the First Baby," *Good Housekeeping,* vol. 193, Oct. 1936, p. 138.

Rudolph H. Dressendorfer, Ph.D., "Physical Training During Pregnancy and Lactation," *The Physician and Sportsmedicine,* vol. 6, no. 2, Feb. 1978, pp. 74–80.

Carol Dilfer, "Jogging Through Pregnancy," *The Jogger,* vol. 8, no. 36, March–April 1976.

Pregnancy and Daily Living, ACOG patient information booklet available free from the ACOG, One East Wacker Drive, Chicago 60601.

ACOG, *Walking During Pregnancy,* ACOG patient information booklet.

CHAPTER 4
TRAVEL

Background for this chapter includes extensive interviews in the travel industry with, among others, medical directors of airlines and passenger ship lines. Of particular importance were interviews with women who traveled during pregnancy. Some material originally appeared in Susan S. Lichtendorf's article on her personal travel experience, which appeared in *The New York Times,* Oct. 24, 1976.

General References

Williams Obstetrics, p. 256.

Kay Lund, "Paving the Way for the Handicapped," United Airlines *Mainliner,* Aug. 1977, p. 74.

ACOG, *Hints for the Pregnant Traveler.*

R. Graeme Cameron, "Should Air Hostesses Continue Flight Duty During the First Trimester of Pregnancy?" *Aerospace Medicine,* May 1973, pp. 552–56.

Paul Scholten, M.D., "Pregnant Stewardess—Should She Fly?" *Space and Environmental Medicine,* Jan. 1976, p. 77.

Immunization During Pregnancy, ACOG Technical Bulletin 20, March 1973.

"Smallpox Vaccination During Pregnancy," *Obstetrics and Gynecology,* Aug. 1975, pp. 223–26.

Hans H. Neumann, M.D., *Foreign Travel Immunization Guide*, 6th ed. (Oradell, N.J.: Medical Economics Book Division, 1977).

R. J. Pepperell, E. Rubenstein, and I. A. Mac Issac, "Motor Car Accidents During Pregnancy," *Obstetrical and Gynecological Survey*, vol. 32, no. 10, Oct. 1977, pp. 659–61.

Safety Belts for People Who Enjoy Living, Pamphlet of the Automobile Association of America.

CHAPTER 5
ACHIEVING A HEALTHY PREGNANCY

General References

Full citations are in notes for Chapter Three.

Williams Obstetrics, pp. 250–55.

Current Obstetric and Gynecologic Diagnosis and Treatment, pp. 237–39.

Précis: An Update in Obstetrics and Gynecology.

Gynecology and Obstetrics: The Health Care of Women.

Nutrition

ACOG Task Force on Nutrition, *Assessment of Maternal Nutrition*, 1978.

ACOG, *Standards for Ambulatory Obstetric Care*, 1974.

ACOG, *Nutrition in Maternal Health Care*, 1974.

Maternal Nutrition and the Course of Pregnancy, U.S. Department of Health, Education and Welfare, reprinted 1975.

Richard W. Wertz and Dorothy C. Wertz, *Lying In: A History of Childbirth in America* (New York: The Free Press, 1977).

Clark Gillespie, M.D., *Your Pregnancy, Month by Month* (New York: Harper and Row, 1977), p. 58.

The point about the need to feed the inner self was made

by Dr. Joan Zuckerberg at The Birth of the American Child Conference, cited in Chapter IX notes.

Material about Weight Watchers International came through interviews with Weight Watcher members, lecturers and the corporation's medical director.

"Fetal and Infant Nutrition and Susceptibility to Obesity," Summary of a workshop sponsored by the Food and Nutrition Board of the National Academy of Sciences, Feb. 1978.

Drugs

Avrin M. Overbach, M.D., and Morton J. Rodman, Ph.D., *Drugs Used with Neonates and During Pregnancy* (Oradell, N.J.: Medical Economics Company Book Division, 1975).

Addictive Drugs and Pregnancy, ACOG Technical Bulletin 21, April 1973.

"Data: Drugs, Alcohol, Tobacco Abuse During Pregnancy," March of Dimes Health Education pamphlet.

Michael Newton, M.D., "On Popping Pills and Potions During Pregnancy," *Family Health/Today's Health,* May 1977.

Alcohol

"Pregnant? Before You Drink, *Think* of Your Unborn Baby," March of Dimes pamphlet.

Jennifer Dunning, "Women Are Warned To Give Up Drinking During Pregnancies," *The New York Times,* June 1, 1977.

"Must Pregnant Women Stop Drinking?" *Medical World News,* June 27, 1977, p. 9.

Cigarette Smoking

J. Kline, Z. Stern, M. Susser, and D. Warburton, "Smoking: A Risk for Spontaneous Abortion," *New England Journal of Medicine,* vol. 297, no. 15, Oct. 13, 1977, pp. 794–96.

"Smoking Held a Primary Factor in Prenatal and Fetal Mortality," *Ob-Gyn News,* vol. 13, no. 19, May 1, 1978, pp. 1 and 27.

Information for this section comes from sources at the American Cancer Society. Reflected in the section are the many studies reported in numerous updates of the U.S. Surgeon General's Report on the hazards of smoking cigarettes, and papers delivered at a 1978 American Cancer Society conference on smoking cessation behavior. These papers included "Women and Smoking: A Realistic Appraisal," by Ellen Gritz, Ph.D., and "How to Reach and Convince Pregnant Women to Give Up Smoking," by Gisela Gastrin, M.D., and Lars M. Ramstrom, Ph.D.

The Environment

Information reflects attendance at a conference of The Scientific Basis for the Public Control of Environmental Health Hazards, presented by the New York Academy of Sciences, June 21–30, 1978. Other references include specific data developed by the March of Dimes for science writers.

CHAPTER 6
THE INNER YOU

Background for this chapter included attendance at The Birth of An American Child Conference on Psychological and Emotional Response to Factors Affecting Pregnancy and Childbirth, Sponsored by the National Institute for the Psychotherapies, May 6, 1978, in New York City. Of particular importance were the following workshops: "Reworking the Delivery Trauma: Postpartum Support Services," led by Jo Ann Magnus, chairperson, Speaker's Bureau of the Mother's Center of the Nassau County Family Service Association, and Patsy Turrini, consultant to the Mother's Center; "Psychological and Psychosomatic Warning Signals Regarding Pregnancy Adaptation," led by Joan Zuckerberg, Ph.D., adjunct assistant professor, Long Island University. Also important were discussions with Tamara Engel of the Jewish Family Service, New York City; Dr. Mary Anna Freidereich, of Rochester,

New York, past president of the American Society for Psychosomatic Obstetrics and Gynecology; Bonnie Donovan of Massachusetts, author of *The Cesarean Birth Experience;* and Dr. Niles Newton.

General References

Aidan MacFarlane, *The Psychology of Childbirth* (Cambridge: Harvard Univ. Press, 1977).

Jean Baker Miller, *Toward a New Psychology of Women* (Boston: Beacon Press, 1976).

Arthur and Libby Colman, *Pregnancy: The Psychological Experience* (New York: Bantam Books, 1977).

Helene Deusch, M.D., *The Psychology of Women,* vol. II, *Motherhood* (New York: Bantam, 1973).

The Boston Women's Health Book Collective, *Our Bodies, Ourselves* (New York: Simon and Schuster, 1971).

Margaret Mead, Ph.D., and Niles Newton, Ph.D., "Cultural Patterning of Perinatal Behaviour," *Childbearing: Its Social and Psychological Aspects,* ed. S. A. Richardson and A. F. Guttmacher (Baltimore: Williams and Wilkins, 1967), pp. 142–230.

Niles Newton, "Emotions of Pregnancy," *Clinical Obstetrics and Gynecology,* vol. 6, no. 3, Sept. 1963, pp. 639–62.

Leonide M. Tanner, "Developmental Tasks of Pregnancy," *Current Concepts in Clinical Nursing,* vol. II, 1969, pp. 292–97.

Ann Belford Ulanov, "Birth and Rebirth: The Effect of an Analyst's Pregnancy on the Transference of Three Patients," *Journal of Analytical Psychology,* vol. 8, no. 2, 1973.

Pauline M. Shereshefsky and Leon J. Yarrow, "Psychological Aspects of a First Pregnancy and Early Postnatal Adaptation," Monograph of the National Institute of Child Health and Human Development (New York: Raven Press, 1973).

Particular References

Judi Thompson, *Healthy Pregnancy the Yoga Way* (New York: Dolphin Books, 1977).

Phyllis Theroux, "Hers," *The New York Times,* Sept. 15, 1977.

Adrienne Rich, *Of Woman Born* (New York: Bantam Books, 1977), pp. 6–7.

H. Heymans and S. T. Winter, "Fears During Pregnancy: Interview Study of 200 Postpartum Women," reprinted in *1977 Year Book of Obstetrics and Gynecology*.

Janie Spelton Weinberg, R.N., M.N., "Body Image Disturbance as a Factor in the Crisis Situation of Pregnancy," *Journal of Obstetrics and Gynecology Nursing,* March/April 1978, pp. 18–20.

Jacqueline Fawcett, Ph.D., "Body Image and the Pregnant Couple," *American Journal of Maternal Child Nursing,* vol. 3, no. 4, July/August 1978, pp. 227–33.

George Schaefer, M.D., *The Expectant Father: A Practical Guide* (Barnes and Noble: Everyday Handbooks, 1972).

Henry Biller, Ph.D., and Dennis Meredith, *Father Power* (New York: Anchor Press, 1975).

Kathryn Antle May, R.N., M.S.N., "Active Involvement of Expectant Fathers in Pregnancy: Some Further Considerations," *Journal of Obstetrics and Gynecology Nursing,* March/April 1978, pp. 7–12.

Cherry Wunderlich, "Expectant Fathers: Recent Research on Their Feelings and Needs," *ICEA News,* Jan. 1977.

Cherry Wunderlich, "Father's Attachment and Adjustment," *ICEA News,* March 1977.

Cherry Wunderlich, "Expectant Fathers: Their Role During Labor and Delivery," *ICEA News,* Feb. 1977.

Jaynelle F. Stichler, Marita S. Bowden, and Elizabeth D. Reimer, "Pregnancy: A Shared Emotional Experience,"

American Journal of Maternal Child Nursing, May/June 1978, pp. 153–57.

Clifford J. Sager, M.D., *Marriage Contracts and Couple Therapy: Hidden Forces in Intimate Relationships* (New York: Brunner, Mazel, 1976).

CHAPTER 7
THE OUTER YOU:
LOOKING GOOD

Development of this chapter included an especially useful interview with David Daines, Davian, New York City, regarding image and appearance. Interviews were also conducted with maternity buyers and fashion coordinators at several major U.S. department stores.

General References

Erving Goffman, *The Presentation of Self in Everyday Life* (Garden City, N.Y.: Anchor Books, 1959).

Erving Goffman, *Encounters: Two Studies in the Sociology of Interaction* (New York: Bobbs-Merrill, 1961).

CHAPTER 8
SEX AND SEXUALITY

Background for this chapter included attendance at the 1977 and 1978 meetings of the Eastern Association for Sex Therapy, and discussions with Dr. Sallie Schumacher of Pittsburgh, past president of EAST; Bryce Britton, a vice-president of Eve's Garden, a sexual boutique for women in New York City; and medical students in Philadelphia who did a survey of sexual attitudes of gynecologists in the metropolitan area.

General References

Lonnie Garfield Barbach, *For Yourself: The Fulfillment of Female Sexuality* (New York: Signet Books, 1976).

Williams Obstetrics, pp. 256–57.

Current Obstetric and Gynecologic Diagnosis and Treatment, pp. 414–19.

Celia J. Falicov, Ph.D., "Sexual Adjustment During First Pregnancy and Post Partum, *American Journal of Obstetrics and Gynecology,* Dec. 1973, pp. 991–1000.

Robert Goodlin, M.D., William Schmidt, and Donald Creeny, M.D., "Uterine Tension and Fetal Heart Rate During Maternal Orgasm," *Obstetrics and Gynecology,* vol. 39, no. 1, Jan. 1972, pp. 125–27.

William Masters and Virginia E. Johnson, *Human Sexual Response* (Boston: Little, Brown, 1966), p. 148.

William E. Pugh, M.D., and Frank L. Fernandez, "Coitus in Late Pregnancy," *Obstetrics and Gynecology,* vol. II, no. 6, Dec. 1953, pp. 636–42.

Nathaniel W. Wagner, Julius C. Butler and Josephine Sanders, "Prematurity and Orgasmic Coitus During Pregnancy: Data on a Small Sample," *Obstetrics and Gynecological Survey,* vol. 32, no. 11, 1977, pp. 697–98, plus related editorial comment.

Robert Goodlin, David W. Keller and Margaret Raffin, "Orgasm in Late Pregnancy," *Obstetrics and Gynecology,* vol. 38, no.6, Dec. 1971, pp. 916–20.

Leon Speroff, M.D., Peter W. Romwell, Ph.D., "Prostaglandins and Reproductive Physiology," *American Journal of Obstetrics and Gynecology,* vol. 107, no. 7, Aug. 1976, pp. 1111–124.

Masters and Johnson, p. 166.

Fritz Fuchs, M.D., and Arnold Klopper, M.D., Ph.D., eds., *Endocrinology of Pregnancy,* 2nd ed. (New York: Harper and Row, 1977), pp. 294–346.

Dr. Fritz Fuchs, "Coitus and Induction of Labor," *Medical Aspects of Human Sexuality,* May 1977, p. 10.

Information about positions was developed from interviews, discussions with sex therapists and material from *More Joy of Sex,* ed. Alex Comfort, M.D., Ph.D. (New York: Simon and Schuster, 1973).

Marvin E. Aronson, M.D., Philip K. Nelson, M.D., "Fatal Air Embolism in Pregnancy Resulting from an Unusual Sex Act," *Obstetrics and Gynecology*, vol. 39, no. 1, Jan. 1967.

"Heat Is on Saunas as Possible Teratogens," *Medical World News*, March 20, 1978.

John Grover, M.D., "Coitus During Pregnancy for Women with a History of Spontaneous Abortion," *Medical Aspects of Human Sexuality*, May 1977, p. 113.

"Happy Mother's Day!" *Hustler*, May 1978.

C. Ford and E. Beach, *Patterns of Sexual Behavior* (New York: Harper and Row, 1951), p. 213–17.

Roman Rechnitz Limner, *Sex and the Unborn Child* (New York: Julian Press, 1969), p. xii.

Sexually Transmitted Disease (STD) Other than Syphilis and Gonorrhea, ACOG technical bulletin, July 1978.

Elizabeth Bing and Libby Colman, *Making Love During Pregnancy* (New York: Bantam Books, 1977), p. 98.

"A Funny Thing Happened on the Way to the Orifice: Women in Gynecology Textbooks," Study by Diane Scully and Pauline Bart of the University of Illinois.

Don A. Solberg, B.A., Julius Butler, M.D., and Nathaniel Wagner, Ph.D., "Sexual Behavior in Pregnancy," *New England Journal of Medicine*, May 24, 1973, pp. 1098–103.

Masters and Johnson, pp. 151–67.

Falicov, p. 997.

Masters and Johnson, p. 167.

Falicov, p. 997.

Niles Newton, Ph.D., "Interrelationship between Sexual Responsiveness, Birth and Breast Feeding," *Contemporary Sexual Behavior: Critical Issues in the 1970's*, ed. Joseph Zubin and John Money (Baltimore: Johns Hopkins University Press, 1973), pp. 77 and 84.

James A. Kenny, Ph.D., "Sexuality of Pregnant and Breastfeeding Women," *Archives of Sexual Behavior,* vol. 2, no. 3, 1973, pp. 215–29.

CHAPTER 9
POSTPARTUM

General References

We have found the following books to be the most helpful in passing through the postpartum and reentry periods:

T. Berry Brazelton, *Infants and Mothers* (New York: Dell, 1972).

T. Berry Brazelton, *Doctor and Child* (New York: Delta, 1978).

Fitzhugh Dodson, *How to Parent* (New York: New American Library, 1971).

Marguerite Kelly and Elia Parsons, *The Mother's Almanac* (Garden City, N.Y.: Doubleday, 1975).

Dr. Benjamin Spock, *Baby and Child Care,* rev. ed. (New York: Pocket Books, 1976).

Burton White, *The First Three Years of Life* (Englewood Cliffs, N.J.: Prentice-Hall, 1965).

Particular References

"Study of New Parents Looks at Impact of Baby's Arrival on the Marriage," *The New York Times,* Jan. 7, 1978, p. 10.

"Parents Help Parents with Newborn Problems," *The New York Times,* Aug. 1, 1978, p. C2.

ABOUT THE AUTHORS

SUSAN S. LICHTENDORF's writing career includes work as a reporter for a New York newspaper, and she is a former science writer for the National Office of the American Cancer Society. Her freelance articles have appeared in newspapers and major national magazines. Currently, she is writing a book about special aspects of women's lives and health. She is a graduate of the City University of New York, and she is a member of the National association of Science Writers.

PHYLLIS L. GILLIS is a freelance writer and contributing editor of *Parents Magazine*. She was formerly a vice president of Louis Harris and Associates and executive director of Gallup International Research Institutes. She has worked as a writer of publications in both Washington and New York. She holds a master of science degree in journalism from the Medill School of Journalism at Northwestern University and a bachelor of arts degree from Michigan State University.

Congratulations— But...

What about all those questions and problems that arrive with a new addition to the family? Here are several invaluable books for any new or expectant mother. They are filled with helpful hints for raising healthy children in a happy home. Best of luck and may all your problems be little ones!

☐	13742	**BETTER HOMES AND GARDENS BABY BOOK**	$2.50
☐	20011	**CARING FOR YOUR UNBORN CHILD** Gots, M.D.'s	$2.95
☐	20340	**UNDERSTANDING PREGNANCY AND CHILDBIRTH** by Sheldon H. Cherry, M.D.	$2.95
☐	14278	**PREGNANCY NOTEBOOK** by Marcia Morton	$2.25
☐	14409	**NINE MONTHS READING** by Robert E. Hall, M.D.	$2.50
☐	12640	**FEED ME! I'M YOURS** by Vicki Lansky	$2.25
☐	14399	**SIX PRACTICAL LESSONS FOR AN EASIER CHILDBIRTH** by Elisabeth Bing	$2.50
☐	20406	**NAME YOUR BABY** by Lareina Rule	$2.50
☐	20432	**YOUR BABY'S SEX: NOW YOU CAN CHOOSE** by Rorvik & Shettles, M.D.'s	$2.50
☐	13901	**THE FIRST TWELVE MONTHS OF LIFE** by Frank Caplan, ed	$2.95
☐	13038	**THE SECOND TWELVE MONTHS OF LIFE** Caplans, eds.	$3.50
☐	14407	**COMPLETE BOOK OF BREASTFEEDING** by M. Eiger, M.D. & S. Olds	$2.50
☐	13711	**IMMACULATE DECEPTION** by Suzanne Arms	$2.95
☐	13895	**PREPARING FOR PARENTHOOD** by Lee Salk	$2.75
☐	12497	**PREGNANCY: THE PSYCHOLOGICAL EXPERIENCE** by Arthur & Libby Colman	$2.25
☐	20149	**MAKING YOUR OWN BABY FOOD** by James Turner	$2.25
☐	13961	**MOVING THROUGH PREGNANCY** by Elisabeth Bing	$2.50
☐	01271	**MAKING LOVE DURING PREGNANCY** Bing & Colman	$6.95

Buy them at your local bookstore or use this handy coupon for ordering:

THE LATEST BOOKS
IN THE BANTAM
BESTSELLING TRADITION

☐	14512	**NO LOVE LOST** Helen van Slyke	$3.75
☐	01328	**TIDES OF LOVE** Patricia Matthews (Large Format)	$5.95
☐	13545	**SOPHIE'S CHOICE** William Styron	$3.50
☐	14200	**PRINCESS DAISY** Judith Krantz	$3.95
☐	20025	**THE FAR PAVILIONS** M. M. Kaye	$4.50
☐	14068	**THE CANADIANS: BLACK ROBE** Robert E. Wall	$2.95
☐	13752	**SHADOW OF THE MOON** M. M. Kaye	$3.95
☐	14249	**CHILDREN OF THE LION** Peter Danielson	$2.95
☐	13980	**TEXAS!** Dana Fuller Ross	$2.75
☐	14968	**THE RENEGADE** Donald Clayton Porter	$2.95
☐	20087	**THE HAWK AND THE DOVE** Leigh Franklin James	$2.95
☐	13641	**PORTRAITS** Cynthia Freeman	$3.50
☐	20670	**FAIRYTALES** Cynthia Freeman	$3.50
☐	14439	**THE EWINGS OF DALLAS** Burt Hirschfeld	$2.75
☐	13992	**CHANTAL** Claire Lorrimer	$2.95

Buy them at your local bookstore or use this handy coupon:

THE FAMILY—TOGETHER AND APART

Choose from this potpourri of titles for the information you need on the many facets of family living.

☐	14211	**LOVE AND SEX IN PLAIN LANGUAGE** Eric W. Johnson	$1.95
☐	14486	**THE PLEASURE BOND** Masters & Johnson	$3.50
☐	20346	**DARE TO DISCIPLINE** J. Dobson	$2.95
☐	13735	**HOW TO SURVIVE YOUR CHILD'S REBELLIOUS TEENS** Myron Brenton	$2.50
☐	14738	**THE PARENT'S BOOK ABOUT DIVORCE** Richard A. Gardner	$3.50
☐	14240	**PREPARING FOR ADOLESCENCE** James Dobson	$2.25
☐	13164	**A PARENT'S GUIDE TO CHILDREN'S READING** Nancy Larrick	$2.50
☐	14731	**P.E.T. IN ACTION** Thomas Gordon with J. Gordon Sands	$3.50
☐	20262	**LOVE AND SEX AND GROWING UP** Johnson & Johnson	$2.25
☐	14232	**THE BOYS AND GIRLS BOOK ABOUT DIVORCE** Richard A. Gardner	$2.25
☐	14572	**HOW TO GET IT TOGETHER WHEN YOUR PARENTS ARE COMING APART** Richards & Willis	$1.95
☐	14768	**ANY WOMAN CAN** David Reuben, M.D.	$2.95
☐	13624	**NAME YOUR BABY** Lareina Rule	$2.25
☐	20078	**OF WOMAN BORN: Motherhood as Experience and Institution** Adrienne Rich	$3.95

Buy them at your local bookstore or use this handy coupon for ordering:

Bantam Books, Inc., Dept. FL, 414 East Golf Road, Des Plaines, Ill. 60016

Please send me the books I have checked above. I am enclosing $_____ (please add $1.00 to cover postage and handling). Send check or money order no cash or C.O.D.'s please.

Mr/Mrs/Miss_____

Address_____

City_____ State/Zip_____

FL—5/81

Please allow four to six weeks for delivery. This offer expires 11/81.